(small)

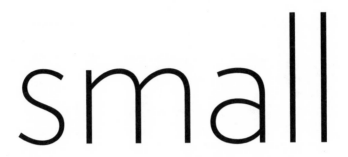

small

Life and Death on the Front Lines
of Pediatric Surgery

CATHERINE MUSEMECHE, MD

DARTMOUTH COLLEGE PRESS
Hanover, New Hampshire

Dartmouth College Press
An imprint of University Press of New England
www.upne.com
© 2014 Catherine Musemeche
All rights reserved
Manufactured in the United States of America
Designed by Eric M. Brooks
Typeset in Whitman by Passumpsic Publishing

For permission to reproduce any of the material
in this book, contact Permissions, University Press of
New England, One Court Street, Suite 250, Lebanon NH
03766; or visit www.upne.com.

Library of Congress Cataloging-in-Publication Data
Musemeche, Catherine, author.
Small: life and death on the front lines of pediatric surgery /
Catherine Musemeche.
    p.; cm.
Includes bibliographical references and index.
ISBN 978-1-61168-442-1 (cloth : alk. paper) —
ISBN 978-1-61168-635-7 (ebook)
I. Title. [DNLM: 1. Surgical Procedures, Operative —
Personal Narratives. 2. Child. 3. General Surgery —
history — Personal Narratives. 4. Infant. 5. Pediatrics —
history — Personal Narratives. WO 925]
RD27.35.B47   617.092 — dc23
[B]   2014014173

5 4 3 2 1

conch

Hold a baby to your ear
As you would a shell:
Sounds of centuries you hear
New centuries foretell.

Who can break a baby's code?
And which is the older —
The listener or his small load?
The held or the holder?

(E. B. WHITE)

contents

introduction

From the beginning, pediatric surgeons had to insist on their very existence at the same time that they were inventing the techniques and tools that would enable them to save the lives of the most vulnerable members of our population, our children. C. Everett Koop stayed late at the hospital filing rubber tubes so they would fit in the tiny airways of premature infants he would operate on the next day. Barbara Barlow, told repeatedly that women had no place in the operating room except as nurses, went on to become the first full-time pediatric surgeon in Harlem and built over one hundred playgrounds along the way. Melvin Smith refused to believe that a baby could not be saved simply because a device to straighten a tiny misshapen chest had not yet been invented.

Those of us who have been fortunate to practice pediatric surgery know that we stand on the shoulders of the giants who came before us in this unheralded field of medicine, men and women without whose perseverance in the face of adversity our specialty would not exist.

I had two goals in writing this book. One was to bring the reader into the operating room, the newborn intensive care unit, the emergency room, and to the bedside to experience what it is like to do this intense, demanding, and sometimes lonely job of a pediatric surgeon. The second was to bring to life the stories of individuals who achieved milestones in the field. While some of these stories are well known in the medical world, others have been buried in the past. All, however, demonstrate the ingenuity and tenacity of surgeons who refused to give up just because a clinical problem seemed next to impossible to solve.

This work is not intended as a comprehensive history of pediatric surgery. It is, rather, one person's attempt to acknowledge some specific accomplishments that demonstrate the courage, persistence, and unselfish devotion one needs to care for sick and injured children — in other words, to be a pediatric surgeon.

"Stitch," I say to the scrub nurse.

I hold out my hand, waiting. Instead of keeping up with me, the next suture ready to slap into my palm, she's hit a snag trying to pull the suture out of the package and load the needle in the gold-handled needle holder. I wish I could reach across the instrument tray and do it myself, but I can't move. If I look away, I'll lose my place, and that will only delay me further. I'm focusing on an area no bigger than a postage stamp through a pair of surgical loupes that magnify my limited view. I can see the exact spot where the next stitch needs to go, between two gaping edges of intestine, the width of a matchstick.

"Let's go," I say. "Let's get this finished."

I know I seem impatient, but it is not because I'm in a hurry to get to something else. My only focus at the moment is on this baby, Clare. I know that every moment she is under the drapes on the operating room table her life is at risk. Born eight weeks early, she weighs only four pounds. A breathing tube no bigger than a straw is keeping her alive during this operation. The correct position of this tube, inside her trachea, is measured in millimeters. If it is accidentally pushed in or pulled out, even a minuscule amount, her lungs will fail to expand and deflate and an alarm will go off.

Any interruption in ventilation will cause us to stop operating. The anesthesiologist will have to check the breathing tube and adjust it as needed. If the tube completely dislodges, the oxygen level in the bloodstream will plummet and within seconds

the baby's heart, deprived of oxygen, will start to slow dangerously. When that happens, the baby will be close to cardiac arrest.
And if her heart does stop beating and normal blood circulation
ceases, not only will this interrupt the operation, it could end it
before we finish repairing the congenital malformation we came
here to fix. We will have to staple everything closed and get out as
quickly as possible.

In other words, a complication like this can result in disaster, a
nightmare for surgeon and patient alike, and I had seen it before.

Three decades ago, when I was training to be a surgeon, I was assisting in an operation to repair bilateral inguinal (groin) hernias,
persistent openings between the lining of the abdomen and the
scrotum, in a premature baby boy with chronic lung disease. This
is normally a straightforward repair that requires making a small
incision on either side of the lower abdomen and locating and
tying off a tissue sac. But on this particular morning, when the pediatric surgeon and I were about to finish and close the skin, the
breathing tube slipped down too far, into the right-side bronchus,
so that only the right lung was being ventilated.

Within seconds, the infant's oxygen level dropped, his heart
rate slowed, and the anesthesiologist disconnected the ventilator and started bagging the baby by hand to inflate his scarred
and stiffened lungs. In his excitement to correct the problem, he
used too much force. The pressure blew out both lungs like they
were dime-store balloons, rendering them temporarily useless.
The chest filled up with air, which compressed the lungs and kept
them from expanding at all.

The surgeon and I pulled off the drapes and started CPR using
two fingers, rather than the weight of an entire hand, to compress
the undersized newborn's heart. Then we incised both sides of
the chest with our scalpels and slid small drainage tubes between
ribs as thin and pliable as Q-tips. Within seconds, the air drained
out of the chest cavity and the tiny lungs reexpanded. The heart

started beating again, and the baby stabilized. We prepped the field and finished closing.

"That's the first time I've ever done bilateral hernias and bilateral chest tubes at the same time," the surgeon said. A nervous laugh spilled out to punctuate his relief.

Everyone in the room knew how close we had come to losing that baby when no one was expecting it. Hernia operations are not usually considered high risk. But because we were working on a baby who weighed four pounds rather than the usual nine, a baby who had been in the neonatal intensive care unit the entire two months of his life and had chronic lung disease, the margin for error was slim enough to be virtually nonexistent.

While pediatric anesthesia has continued to improve since this case took place, similar mishaps can still occur. Pediatric patients, particularly infants, have shorter, smaller-diameter airways compared to the larger anatomical structures of adults. With infants it takes only a slight imprecision to throw everything into chaos — a breathing tube that slid in too far or not far enough, too much pressure used to inflate the lungs, the slightest bit of swelling in the lining of the bronchus. What appears on the surface to be a tiny error can cause the vital signs to destabilize, the monitors to alarm, the eruption of a full-out emergency where utter calm had reigned only moments before.

There is no such thing as a routine operation in a baby.

As I wait for the scrub nurse to hand me the next suture, all the things that can go wrong run through my mind: the breathing tube, Clare's temperature, whether the closure will leak or close off from scarring because the sutures are too far apart or too close together. *Does she need another dose of antibiotics? More blood? Will she get a postop infection? Pneumonia? Will the whole thing fall apart and have to be done over again?*

These passing seconds seem like a long time, long enough for me to wonder if there were any way to avoid the delay, long enough to think about exactly how I will line up the stitch again should I lose my place, long enough to remind myself that I am, after all, simply waiting in this 80-degree cauldron, baking under radiant warmers like a carton of French fries on the back counter of a McDonald's. The heat is necessary to keep the baby warm, but consequently sweat is starting to drip down my back under the impermeable layers of my gown. At least for now, though, the baby is stable. The price of this wait so far, measured in time, not disaster.

The situation could be much worse. The baby could be moving, seizing, crashing, or bleeding. But, still, all I want at this moment is for the next stitch to be placed perfectly into my hand, now. Otherwise, I will have to stand here, bent over, peering into this tiny body cavity, the muscles between my shoulder blades knotted and tightening down, doing nothing whatsoever to finish this operation that must be completed before catastrophe strikes.

Operating is not an individual event. It is a team effort.

I need an operating room, the right equipment, a pediatric anesthesiologist, a scrub tech, a circulating nurse, and on some days another surgeon to assist. I have to rely on other people in this high-pressure venue, people I do not always choose, people who may not be as torqued up as I am when I'm operating on a premature infant, people who may not fully appreciate what is at stake.

The nurses and techs assigned to my room may be inexperienced in neonatal operations and may have only been assigned at the last minute because the regular scrub tech is sick or because it's a holiday, night, or weekend and everyone else has gone home. They might be slow, inexperienced, and unaware of the risk of imprecision and delays.

And then I am stuck sweating this out with an assistant who cannot anticipate my next move, who runs out of suture at a critical time, who does not have a single, necessary, 6-zero prolene on an RB needle, loaded and ready to pass so I can put in the next stitch. These are not idle minutes. They are minutes that add risk, something I can't take the time to explain.

I don't have the ideal team every day, but I still have to get the case done as safely as possible. I have a baby's future in my hands, and I have to perform.

Every baby makes a lengthy journey to get to this place we call "life," but they don't all show up ready for it when they arrive. Organs are formed through a complicated set of maneuvers that take place from the third to the eighth weeks of gestation, a critical period for normal development.[1] First, cells must follow orders to replicate, head one direction or the other, or simply disappear. Then, groups of cells have to come together and fold into a certain shape, like origami, to make something like a heart or a liver. The more intricate the intended organ function, the more precise and directed the folding must be to avoid an inadvertent malformation.

To form a perfect baby, this must happen many times over. If a miscue occurs during this vulnerable period of an embryo's development, a part could turn out to be defective, like a malfunctioning thermostat in an expensive German sedan. The rest of the superbly designed engine can be perfectly tuned, but if that one essential part isn't working, the car is going to overheat, and it won't be long before it stops running altogether.

Congenital malformations, or "birth defects," occur in approximately 3 percent of infants in the United States[2] and are responsible for a quarter of infant deaths.[3]

Families invariably ask, "Why did this happen to our baby?"

This question is the one that lingers most when an abnormality appears. Long after a diagnosis is made and an operation is performed, variations of the question recur. *What caused this? What did we do wrong?*

Parents always want to fault themselves when their children are suffering. *Is it something we overlooked during the pregnancy? A vitamin not taken? A fall? A virus? Which side of the family did this come from? Is it something inherited from an odd-looking cousin twice removed?*

No matter how the query is framed or how many different ways we examine the situation or suggest clues, in the majority of cases the answer will be the same.

We don't know.

In 40 to 45 percent of cases, the cause of a birth defect is unknown. In about one-third a genetic abnormality, an error in the DNA, is the cause, due to either a recognized chromosomal abnormality, like cystic fibrosis or sickle cell disease, or a spontaneous gene mutation such as Down syndrome. In a small number of cases, only 3 percent, a close examination of the prenatal course will reveal an in utero exposure to an external or environmental agent that can affect the development of a fetus, such as alcohol, drugs, or a virus (e.g., rubella). And in about a quarter of cases genetics and the environment combine in misguided ways to throw off normal development.[4]

Chromosomes are tricky beasts, each one made up of thousands of genes. I got my first whiff of just how complicated they were when I came close to flunking a genetics course in college. We worked endless problems trying to figure out what would happen to a developing embryo when different sections of chromosomes broke apart and clumsily reattached slightly askew — that is, when the normal forty-six chromosomes (twenty-three from each parent) went off script. Scrambling a future human's genetic code is like trying to bake a cake with ingredients that are mixed in randomly and in the wrong proportions. You can bet something's not going to turn out right — the cake might be flat, taste too salty, or be so dry it sticks to the roof of your mouth — but you won't know exactly how off it will be until it comes out of the oven.

Chromosomes provide instructions to a person's entire body, every single cell. Each directive gets broadcast system wide, like hitting the "reply all" button. A seeming blip of misinformation can have a huge impact and mean the difference between a typical life accomplishing routine tasks and a challenged existence in a body with malformed organs, intellectual challenges, and an appearance that is off, just enough that everyone notices.

Even the slightest chromosomal defect, a minute interruption in the genetic code, can be devastating to normal development. There are about a million ways for the sperm/egg merger to end in disaster, and approximately 50 percent of conceptions end in spontaneous abortion.[5] At least half of these miscarried fetuses do, in fact, have major chromosomal abnormalities. This makes chromosomal disorders some of the most common and lethal afflictions of mankind. A chromosomal abnormality will be present in one in two hundred live births.[6]

A chromosome anomaly known as a trisomy occurs when there are three copies of a particular chromosome, instead of the usual two. Sometimes when an entire chromosome is gained or lost, as with trisomy 16 or trisomy 22, the result is universally fatal. Other trisomies, such as trisomy 21, are survivable because the chromosome itself has fewer genes and therefore impacts fewer physical traits. Commonly known as Down syndrome, trisomy 21 is one of the most common chromosomal defects, occurring in up to one in every eight hundred live births.

Genetic disorders like Tay-Sachs or sickle cell might be passed down through the family tree by carriers. Other defects come out of nowhere, a spontaneous mutation in a chromosome's genetic material caused by a random event. One can only guess at the cause. *Was the egg too old? Radiation damage to the ovary or testicles somewhere along the line? In utero drug or alcohol exposure?* Most of the time the inciting event will never be uncovered, but that doesn't stop the endless circle of speculation—and sometimes even the pinning of blame on oneself or one's partner—that invariably ensues.

Like crime scene detectives arriving after the fact, surgeons can reconstruct a developmental sequence based on the evidence left behind—a hole that should have closed or should have stayed open, a membrane that didn't form, structures that failed to separate or failed to fuse. Beyond that, it is difficult to pinpoint a specific factor that caused most embryologic detours.

Pediatric surgeons train for a decade to be able to recognize and correct congenital malformations. Before we ever see a baby, another physician, usually a neonatologist, relays the medical history, a very short story in the case of a newborn. Our minds immediately start to work assembling the key words from the neonatologist. We make a list, the differential diagnosis, of all the possible causes of the baby's symptoms. We rank them in order of probability.

Before we ever examine the infant or look at her X-rays, we already have in mind the top three causes of throwing up green-colored liquid or a distended abdomen, bloody stools, or choking and turning blue with the first feeding. Everything we do next—a physical exam, imaging studies, and lab tests—is aimed at gathering the information we need to narrow the list and funnel the data toward a single right answer, the diagnosis.

Operating on a baby to correct a congenital anomaly, many of which occur only once in every 2,500 to 5,000 live births, is not as straightforward as removing a diseased appendix or gallbladder. Even though there is a pattern to most surgically correctible congenital anomalies, there may be variations of a particular disorder, and an experienced pediatric surgeon will be looking for them. For example, if a baby has one blockage in the intestine, up to 10 percent of such babies could have more blockages, and the entire intestine must be inspected to find them. The diagnosis of a particular type of congenital abnormality may be an indication that there are also others. When a baby is born with a connection between the trachea and the esophagus, a surgeon must examine and study the infant for abnormalities of the vertebrae, anus, heart, kidneys, and limbs, because a condition known as the VACTERL syndrome is present in up to 25 percent of babies with the trachea-esophageal connection.

Other conditions seem like they should be anatomically simple to repair yet can still be fatal. Diaphragmatic hernia, a condition where there is a hole in the muscular diaphragm that separates the abdominal cavity from the thoracic cavity, is a good example. Technically, the hole is relatively easy to patch or close, but because it allows the intestines to slip into the chest during the first trimester of pregnancy, the lungs are compressed and fail to develop normally. Instead of being born with two full lungs, these babies are born with one lung and only a tiny, underdeveloped nubbin of another. The lungs need to be supported until the babies are stable and on low ventilator settings, and the operation may have to be put on hold. Approximately half the babies born with this deceptively simple defect will not have sufficient lung tissue to survive and will die of lung failure in the first week of life. Closing the hole in the diaphragm will not save them.

There is no such thing as a routine operation, because there is more to pediatric surgery than learning how to cut and sew in miniature. The basic skills of operating—making incisions, tying knots, understanding how to repair and reconnect organs—are the same no matter what the size of the patient. But our patients aren't just smaller; they are fragile and complicated in ways that increase the risk.

Infants are not just small adults. The first twenty-eight days of life encompass the most dramatic physiological changes seen in humans.[7] Newborns have a more flexible chest wall, and the amount of air they can take in is limited. The respiratory rate of 30–50 is roughly triple that of adults. The resting newborn heart rate (120–160 beats per minute) is approximately twice that of adults. Neonates have a higher ratio of body surface area to body weight than adults, increasing the potential area through which body heat can be lost. Seventy-five percent of neonatal body weight is water, compared to 60 percent for adults, and thus neonates are subject to becoming dehydrated rapidly. Organs such as the kidneys and liver are not completely mature and are inefficient at filtering toxins. Drug doses have to be carefully calculated, and some drugs must be avoided altogether.

The physiologic differences compared to adults are especially true of the 12 percent of newborns who are born prematurely, babies less than thirty-seven weeks gestation who have underdeveloped organs that may not function normally at birth. Those who are just a few weeks early may escape with no complications, but the more premature, the more prone an infant is to developing one or more life-threatening complications.

An extremely premature newborn, one born at twenty-two to twenty-five weeks gestation, just over half a normal pregnancy, may weigh as little as a pound. These are the smallest human beings alive. As small as kittens, they can fit in the palm of your hand. Their veins are visible beneath translucent tissue-paper skin. Pliable ears fold over and stick to the sides of oversized heads crowned with wispy hair. Because they are deficient in subcutaneous fat, their skin hangs loose from their Barbie-doll arms and legs.

They are too premature to control their own body temperatures, too tiny to eat, too weak to breathe. They live in incubators like aquarium-bound fish, where we feed them through toothpick-sized tubes inserted into stomachs as small as walnuts, inflate their gauzy butterfly-shaped lungs, and pour antibiotics into spiderweb veins.

These unfinished humans face numerous challenges as they struggle to survive outside the womb. Because of their underdeveloped brains they are subject to apnea (periods during which breathing stops for twenty seconds or longer), difficulty sucking and swallowing normally, and a complication known as intraventricular hemorrhage, a type of bleeding into the part of the brain where the cerebrospinal fluid is produced, which, when severe, can cause profound neurologic disability.

They develop respiratory distress because the air sacs to their lungs are not fully developed. Their small stomachs empty slowly, and because their gastrointestinal tract is so immature, they are subject to developing necrotizing enterocolitis, a disease that inflames the intestine and can cause portions of it to die. They are less able to clear waste products from the bloodstream due to their underdeveloped kidneys and liver. They are prone to low blood sugar, lose heat rapidly, and have decreased antibody levels in the bloodstream, leading to an increased risk of a potentially fatal bloodstream infection.

These tiniest of humans are not ideal candidates for any kind of operation, but in times of life-threatening emergency, we are forced to cut them open, knowing that each trip to the operating room traumatizes their fragile bodies. Their organs are like Jell-O and barely hold together when our imposing adult fingers push and pull. We patch what can be salvaged, taking out dead and malformed pieces. When we are short of parts, we rearrange and make do, aware that we might have to come back and reshuffle later. Then we sew it all back together with a needle the size of an eyelash that grips mere slivers of muscle.

Clare was born about two months early. On the outside she is a fully formed replica of a term infant at about half the usual size, but she vomits everything she sucks down. An upper GI (a barium X-ray that outlines the anatomy of the upper gastrointestinal tract) has confirmed the diagnosis of duodenal atresia, a blockage in the first part of the intestine called the duodenum. The food she takes in cannot move past it.

Like most structural defects, there is no known cause for this aberration in development. Early in gestation, the sixth week, the intestine is a solid tube.[8] A few weeks later it hollows out through a process known as recanalization to open the passage for food. If this process fails or if the blood vessels to the intestine are compromised, a blockage or atresia may result.[9] Like a highway that ends abruptly in a cul-de-sac, anything the baby eats will back up until a new connection is created. To repair this, she will need a major operation under general anesthesia.

The thought of it terrifies her parents. They are upper middle class, well-educated, and appropriately concerned. Their other children are healthy, and they had no warning during pregnancy that something might be wrong with Clare, their fourth. They never imagined that their baby might be in an operating room on the second day of life.

I operate on babies like Clare every day, many at much higher risk because of diseased hearts or lungs. No matter what the risk, it's personal, and her parents will be desperately anxious until we're done.

At the very minimum I will need to explain the operation in enough detail for the parents to understand how I will repair their daughter's condition. I want to tell them each step, disclose all the risks, but they are still absorbing the news. If I give them too much information, they'll be overwhelmed. If I don't give them enough, they won't be able to give informed consent, which, by law, is required.

The night before the operation I sit with them in the neonatal intensive care unit (NICU) waiting room on worn plaid couches donated by the women's auxiliary, dimly lit by cheap ceramic lamps. I draw pictures, write out unfamiliar words, answer questions. But how much can they really understand about conditions so unusual it has taken me years to understand them myself? I have to tell them enough so that two things would be clear. They have to appreciate the real risk involved, and they need to trust that I know what I'm doing.

The next day I make a two-inch incision on the right side of Clare's abdomen and peer inside at a crowded landscape, looking for familiar structures like a named exit on a highway to point me in the right direction. First I have to move the pale glistening tubules of intestine out of the way so that I can get down to the duodenum, the area that is blocked. I pick up the colon and dissect it off to the side, and the dilated obstructed duodenum comes into view. The pancreas and bile ducts are nearby, and care must be taken to avoid them and an array of crisscrossing blood vessels in this area.

The first part of the intestine, the duodenum, closest to the stomach, has enlarged during gestation from the accumulated intestinal secretions. It is now three times the normal size, as large as an adult thumb. The other end that connects to the rest of the intestine is much harder to find. It is buried even deeper beneath the obstructed portion. Eventually I find the blind-ending tube, half the width of a pencil, thin and fragile. Just picking it up with forceps can crush the delicate layers.

Now I have the two ends of the first part of the intestine that need to be joined together. Because of the size discrepancy between the two ends, the reconnection must be performed with absolute precision so that there are no gaps between the sutures. I make an incision in each one and line up the two openings with tacking sutures, preparing to sew the intestine together. By the time I'm finished, the stitches have to be close enough to ensure a watertight seal, but not so close that they constrict the outflow through the tube-shaped intestine that is only millimeters in diameter at best.

I use the finest suture available, as thin as a strand of hair, to sew first the back wall of the intestine, like the inside of a pipe, and then work my way around to the front. It is here where I have to pause and wait for the scrub nurse to hand me the stitch and ruminate at length about all the possible complications. Eventually I put in eight sutures and tie each one individually. Next comes the squish test: gently milking liquid through the connection with my fingers to see that it is patent and looking for bubbles at the suture line that might suggest a leak. The connection appears secure. If the tissues heal according to plan, baby Clare should be able to eat in about a week.

After the operation we pack Clare into a temperature-controlled, see-through isolette and transport her back to the NICU. I meet her parents there and stand next to them at their baby's bedside. Nurses, respiratory therapists, and neonatologists swarm the bed. One person is drawing blood. Another is connecting the ventilator. Someone else is starting fluids and medications. Monitors incite a chorus of beeps and bells at the slightest irregularity in vital signs. It is hard to even see the baby under the nest of tubes and lines attached to her.

"It looks a little crazy," I begin, "but this is routine for a big operation. We need all these tubes and monitors to keep her safe while she heals. One by one, as she gets better, they'll start to disappear."

I am trying to construct a narrative that can explain, disclose, comfort, and encourage all at the same time. The parents earnestly scan my face, waiting to hear the words that will bring them back to earth, to the normal life they vacated when this nightmare began.

I learned the operations years ago. Finding the right words, knowing what to say when, has taken me longer. Composing them in just the right way is as important to these parents as anything else I have done all day, as essential as the thread of life that binds baby Clare together.

bunny rabbits, boston, and babies

Never underestimate the capacity of a peripheral nerve to retain IV fluid.

These are the words I hear in my head as I bend over a baby's leg, straightening it, taping it down, and prepping it with Betadine swabs. This internal coach, the voice of my former chief of surgery, is neither random nor imagined. He had a way of tucking these instructive sound bites within the impressionable folds of a trainee's brain — not necessarily a gentle process, but one that made them more memorable. Years later, his words remind me that structures that have the same size, color, and longitudinal orientation as veins may, in fact, be something else. They may be nerves or tendons, structures that have very different purposes than veins and are best left undisturbed in a baby's leg.

Like a kicker who lines up a field goal the same way for each attempt, I feel the femoral pulse in the baby's groin and drop down a centimeter before making my quarter-inch incision directly over the presumed location of the saphenous vein. My habitual maneuvers don't guarantee success, but surgeons, understanding that skill will only take you so far, carry the burden of superstition into each operation. They cling to ritual, performing each step of a procedure in the exact same sequence every time so that nothing important is skipped.

I tease apart globules of subcutaneous fat with a needle-nose mosquito hemostat, the smallest clamp made, being careful not to stray into the translucent fibers of the thigh muscle underneath. The elusive thread of the saphenous vein runs the length of the leg starting just in front of the medial malleolus, the ankle bone, on the inside surface of the lower leg, where in thin patients you can see it and run your finger down its sinewy contour. The vein tracks up the lower leg straight up to the knee, then angles off through the thigh to the groin, where it dives into the deeper reservoir of the femoral vein.

Decades from now, some heart surgeon somewhere might use this same vein to bypass the clogged and calcified coronary arteries of this patient. This could be the vein that sends her, in middle age, to a plastic surgeon to ream out unsightly swellings known as varicosities. This very vein might one day become inflamed, advancing to a painful case of phlebitis, and cause her to call in sick to work.

But before those trials will ever have a chance to materialize, this premature infant, with fledgling lungs that require ventilator support, must grow up and mature into adulthood. She must first survive this hospitalization and the danger of having been introduced to the world as an incomplete human vulnerable to disease, infection, and disability. That means finding a vein.

It sounds like a simple task: finding a vein and inserting an IV. It's the kind of chore that surely someone other than a surgeon could perform. And that is the case for most adults who require an IV. But the veins of adults are garden hoses — bigger, obvious, thicker, and more durable compared to the fragile channels of premature infants. Getting an IV started in a tiny baby is not a given. It is a gift, acquired with skill, experience, and patience.

There are times when the frontline nurses, nurse practitioners, and neonatologists have all tried and failed to get an IV started. The pediatric surgeon is then called in, the last resort, obliged to work where others have tread before on bruised arms and legs peppered with crusted-over needle sticks from failed attempts. A surgeon is trained to have the skills to delve deeper, cut beneath the skin, and find a vein when no one else can.

But that doesn't mean it will be easy.

"The ratio of congenital absence of the saphenous vein is inversely proportional to the experience of the surgeon," leading pediatric surgeon Dr. Willis Potts once noted.[1] In other words, a surgeon who couldn't find the vein might be prone to blaming the failure on an anatomic anomaly rather than his own limited technical skill. Maybe the vein just wasn't located where it was supposed to be. Potts made the statement in the 1950s, an era when a surgical procedure known as a "cut-down" was frequently required before undertaking a major operation. A cut-down is a method of starting an IV that requires an incision in the skin and dissection of a length of vein in which to directly insert an IV catheter. For patients who have had multiple IVs in the past, getting the IV started might require more time and energy than the operation itself.

The relentless chirping of an unanswered pager, a signal that emergencies are piling up around the hospital, interrupts my concentration, but everything else will have to wait. Nothing matters more than what is happening in this dime-sized area that I'm focused on now and getting to know better with each passing minute.

I must find this vein.

I stand up straight and ask the nurse to adjust the headlight I wear tightened around my head like a ceremonial crown and the loupes built into my glasses that magnify tiny structures. The nurse tunes the radio to a country station. I palm the hemostat and start spreading again. It's got to be here somewhere. I spread more toward the right, then the left. I move up a millimeter and back down another and suddenly, a ribbon of purple bobs in a sea of yellow.

"Is that it?" the nurse asks, disappointment wrinkling her brow as she leans over my shoulder and inspects the ridiculously small strand I've lassoed with a suture.

I don't blame her for thinking this will never work, that I'll never be able to create an opening in the vein without cutting it in

two, and if I do manage to open it without destroying it, the catheter will never fit. I pick up a pointed 11 blade, sharp side turned
up, and flick it halfway across the width of the vein. The hole is so
small I can barely imagine where it might be.

ivs are just one moving part of the clockwork necessary to care for
a hospitalized child. They are the lifelines for treatment, conduits
for intravenous fluids, medications, and even nutrition when babies can't eat for days. When they are in place and working well,
they should recede into the background, just another piece of institutional scenery, like a heart monitor mounted on a wall.

But when an iv is difficult to maintain or can't be started at all,
for instance when a baby has been sick a long time and all visible veins have been used, the need to find a vein rises to the top
of the day's priority list. Restorative fluids can't be infused into
a dehydrated baby without one. A septic child will miss a dose
of powerful antibiotics while bacteria spread unchecked in the
bloodstream. The vital signs of a baby with a cardiac defect will
slump without the support of drugs to strengthen his heartbeat.

If there is no working iv, the plan of care grinds to a halt.

In *The Surgery of Infancy and Childhood*, published in 1953, the tedious task of starting and maintaining ivs in babies and small children is portrayed in a series of dramatic photographs.[2] In the first,
a child undergoing an intravenous infusion is turned on her side,
fixed in this position with four-point restraints, ankles and arms
strapped to the rails of her bed.

"Sedation is essential," the legend reads.

In the next, a primitive technique of inserting a needle into
the scalp vein of a baby's shaved head is demonstrated. The head
is wedged between sandbags in the crib to limit movement as the
baby is kept flat on his back, unable to move, unable to eat or
drink. "With luck, the needle will stay in place for 12–18 hours,"
the author advises.

And, in perhaps the most surreal example of the practice of the time, an infant lies swaddled and strapped down, needles impaled in each thigh as if to stake him to the table. Mirror-image sections of rubber tubing snake away from his legs and merge at a Y-connector like feeder lanes dumping into a highway overpass.

In the 1950s, before the existence of the multitude of devices and materials used in medicine today, steel needles were used to infuse intravenous fluids into patients.[3] Steel was a good choice because it could be heat sterilized, was durable, and would maintain a rigid shape without bending. Hollow steel needles are still used today for injecting tissue, a well-suited purpose, as their razor-sharp tips can easily penetrate the skin, fat, and muscle of the human body. But those same qualities posed a hazard when they were used as intravenous catheters in the veins of children. The bevel, or tip of the needle, could easily lacerate their small-caliber, thin-walled veins, causing extravasation, a leaking of fluid out of the vein and into surrounding tissues.

The slightest movement by a child, such as kicking a leg or bending an elbow, could cause dislodgement of the needle, the correct position of which was measured in fractions of a millimeter in a vein that had the caliber of a pencil lead. This movement could cause the needle to leak into the tissues around the vein. If anything other than intravenous fluids was infusing at the time (e.g., antibiotics or calcium), the fluid leaking out could cause severe chemical irritation, leading to infection and sloughing of the surrounding skin and subcutaneous tissue. The risks of either losing the iv or injuring the patient therefore mandated that a child be kept as still as possible even when that appeared inhumane.

Despite near complete immobilization, ivs would seldom last more than a day or two. If a child needed ivs for a week or more, it wasn't long before every available vein in the body—hands, arms, feet, legs, neck, and scalp—was used up. The only remaining option to find a vein was to perform a small operation, a cut-down.

In the worst-case scenario, when the supply of veins had been exhausted by all available means, physicians were forced to get by without one. They could give medications by intramuscular injection, but the last resort for administering fluids without an IV was hypodermoclysis, a method of injecting fluid under the skin (still used today by veterinarians). If a large amount of fluid was injected all at once, it could raise a visible protrusion as big as a grapefruit that would hang off the child's back or thigh. Fluids could only be infused slowly, absorption was unpredictable, and wound complications from skin irritation were common.[4]

Throughout the 1940s and '50s, at the same time pediatric surgeons were struggling with maintaining steel needles in babies' veins, they were striving to crack through the shell of general surgery and develop a distinct specialty devoted to the surgery of children.

Dr. C. Everett Koop, who would later become surgeon general of the United States under President Ronald Reagan, arrived at the Children's Hospital of Philadelphia (CHOP) in 1947. He had just finished his pediatric surgical training at the prestigious Boston Children's Hospital with the founding giants of the specialty, Dr. William Ladd and Dr. Robert Gross. On arrival, Koop was the only trained pediatric surgeon in Pennsylvania and the first surgeon-in-chief at the oldest children's hospital in the country. Koop was eager to get to work, yet he sat for hours in the library with nothing to do.[5] Even though there were children on the wards who needed operations and were dying without them, the pediatricians would not call him.[6]

How had Koop gotten himself into this predicament, taking a job at a hospital where no one would refer patients to him, where he was so disrespected that he was not even assigned an office?

Pediatric surgery had not been his first choice. He was planning to become a cancer surgeon until he met with Dr. I. S. Ravdin, the chief of surgery at the University of Pennsylvania, to discuss his future. Ravdin unveiled a different plan.[7]

There had been a recent mishap at the children's hospital. A delay in performing a simple operation had resulted in a child's death. Following an uprising by the nursing staff, Ravdin picked Koop to go to Boston to train in pediatric surgery. Ravdin dictated that Koop would then return to Philadelphia, bringing with him the expertise to start a pediatric surgery program.

"My mind was flooded with doubts," Koop would later recall about his decision to accept Ravdin's offer.[8] With the exception of a few lectures on feeding infants, pediatrics had been omitted from his medical school curriculum. When World War II started, his internship was shortened and the pediatrics rotation was cut. He'd had no pediatric surgery rotation during his residency. He had seen only three newborn operations as a resident, and one of them was "botched."[9] It was an era when doctors were afraid to put children under anesthesia for fear they would be unable to wake them up.

The career risk of training to become a pediatric surgeon was unsettling. Ravdin was asking Koop to commit to a field he knew little about, a specialty that did not appear to have much of a future. Koop was not even sure he would be busy enough to support his family. He was not familiar with the methods of diagnosis for pediatric patients, the operations, or the postoperative care, but with doubts in hand he headed up to Boston to train with the two founding fathers of pediatric surgery, Dr. Ladd and Dr. Gross. Boston Children's Hospital was the epicenter of pediatric surgery in the 1940s and '50s.

Before World War I, Dr. Ladd had worked in hospitals around Boston primarily as a general surgeon, but he had also volunteered at the Boston Children's Hospital, doing mostly charity cases.[10] In 1917 Ladd was part of an American Red Cross Unit that was dispatched from Boston to Halifax, Nova Scotia, after a French munitions vessel, the *Mont Blanc*, had exploded. The explosion flattened the city and injured thousands, many of whom were children.[11] Between volunteering at the children's hospital and working with the Halifax disaster victims, Ladd discovered a passion for taking care of children. As "soon as it was feasible" after the war, he devoted himself exclusively to performing pediatric surgery at the Boston Children's Hospital, where he served as surgeon-in-chief from 1927 to 1945.[12]

Ladd's most famous trainee during those years was Robert Gross, who served as his chief resident in 1938. Gross, who studied pathology for two years prior to beginning his surgical training, had a uniquely broad foundation in human anatomy. This preparation served him well as a surgeon who devised new operations. He became particularly interested in congenital heart disease and focused on developing a technique to close off an abnormal connection between the heart and the aorta—a patent ductus arteriosus—that, if not corrected, inevitably led to heart failure. He tested out his techniques for closure in the autopsy room and the animal lab, and while Ladd was on vacation in Europe he performed the first successful ligation of a patent ductus arteriosus on a seven-year-old girl.[13]

This was only the first of numerous novel operations attributed to Gross throughout his career, one that solidified his recognition as the "father of pediatric surgery." But he paid a price for his precocious correction of the first patent ductus arteriosus. Ladd never forgave Gross for carrying out the procedure without his knowledge, and when it came time to appoint Ladd's successor at the Boston Children's Hospital, the heir apparent was forced to wait two years.[14]

Koop was not the only young surgeon to experience career doubts. In 1951 a young Alex Haller, who would later become chief of pediatric surgery at Johns Hopkins University, expressed a desire to become a pediatric surgeon to Dr. Alfred Blalock, the chief of surgery. "I'm not sure there is a future for a specialty of children's surgery," Blalock said.[15] Another mentor advised him that he might not be able to make a living operating only on children and that he should let pediatric surgery be his "hobby."[16]

Koop had further reservations about being viewed as a brash young upstart purporting to introduce an entirely new branch of surgery to Philadelphia. Because of medical advances made during World War II, orthopedic surgery and plastic surgery were already branching off from general surgery. Koop knew that another new specialty that would further "splinter the log" of general surgery, siphoning cases away from adult general surgeons, was distinctly unwelcome. Adult general surgeons and anatomic specialists such as ear, nose, and throat surgeons and urologists had no intention of surrendering territory to a new specialty designed to carve out a swath of their existing patient base based on age. The prevailing attitude was that operating on children was a scaled-down version of operating on adults.

No special skills were thought to be required.

"All of us had exactly the same problems in getting started — hostility from the medical community but especially from the surgeons," Koop later recalled. "A prominent surgeon once told Ladd that anyone who could operate on a bunny rabbit could operate on newborns."[17]

In reality, though, babies with surgically correctable conditions all too often died for lack of a trained pediatric surgeon who knew how to repair them. When they did, according to Haller, excuses such as the baby was "too little to live" or "this was God's will" were made.[18]

It was a predicament that Dr. Willis Potts, the head of pediatric surgery at Children's Memorial Hospital in Chicago, lamented in his 1954 address to the Institute of Medicine. "Children's surgery has been forgotten," he said, noting that in the forty-five then existing children's hospitals in the country, all were staffed by "first-class" pediatricians, but only eight had surgical services headed up by full-time pediatric surgeons.[19] He went on to delineate the qualifications that distinguished pediatric surgeons from general surgeons and how taking care of children was different from adults.

"An operation done on a 150 pound adult is not divided by a factor of 15 when one is operating on a 10 pound child," he said.[20] Sick children breathed rapidly. Their temperatures were labile. They lost body heat in the operating room and could succumb to hypothermia. They had increased fluid requirements and a narrow margin between good health and death. A sick child had to be monitored closely; he could look stable one minute and be dead an hour later.

Young children were reticent to speak in the company of strangers and were not going to announce their symptoms. This mandated that pediatric surgeons study and observe their patients for clues to diagnosis. Toddlers would complain of belly pain when in reality they had a sore throat or pneumonia. A ten-day-old infant would unmistakably express nausea by opening his mouth and moving his tongue as if to spit something out. Whimpering was a sign that a child was in danger of an early death. Screaming showed vigor and portended a favorable outcome.

The origins and treatment of surgical ills in children were often completely foreign compared to adults. When an adult presented with rectal bleeding, it was most likely caused by hemorrhoids or colon cancer. The very same symptom presenting in a child would likely be due to entirely different conditions, such as a Meckel's diverticulum (a congenital pouch that hangs off the wall of the small intestine that can become ulcerated), an anal fissure, or a rectal polyp.

Babies in particular were subject to rare congenital anomalies, conditions such as imperforate anus, a complete absence of the rectum, or a tracheoesophageal fistula, an abnormal connection of the esophagus and the trachea. How could an adult specialist who had never seen such conditions be expected to treat them? Pediatric surgeons, working in children's hospitals where they focused solely on treating babies and children, would become familiar with these unusual conditions and gain sufficient expertise to enable the successful treatment of congenital anomalies.[21]

When Koop finished his training in Boston and returned to CHOP, he was greeted at the door by a pediatric resident and told he wasn't wanted and should go back where he came from.[22] The pediatricians were accustomed to being in charge without any full-time surgeons to get in their way. They controlled referrals and determined what cases Koop would get. They were satisfied with the status quo: a group of four general surgeons who covered the hospital part time, dropping by to operate only when absolutely necessary and then turning the patients back over to the pediatricians. The presence of Koop, a full-time pediatric surgeon intent on building a program, threatened their control. To complicate matters further, the party line was that the risk of surgery was prohibitively high in infants and children and should only be undertaken as a last resort.

There was no denying that the risk of surgery for infants and children was greater compared to adults. Pediatric patients had smaller blood volumes and less physiologic reserve, and the risks of anesthesia were considerably higher, all of which led to increased postoperative complications and high mortality.

Operating on children had to be viewed as a safe option if referrals were going to increase, but that wouldn't happen without advances in techniques and equipment, expertise that could not be developed in a void.

One of the first hurdles that had to be overcome for pediatric surgery to be successful as a specialty was the inherent danger in putting a child under anesthesia. Koop himself was "horrified" at what passed as anesthesia when he first arrived at CHOP.[23] A nurse anesthetist would hang a curved tube in the corner of the mouth of a child, infuse ether vapor through it, and leave the room to start another case. It is difficult to imagine that a child's vital signs and airway were not more closely monitored while under anesthesia, but this was standard operating procedure at one of the best children's hospitals of the day.

Much to Koop's relief, anesthesiologist Dr. Margery "Margo" Deming, who had been dispatched to the Children's Hospital of Los Angeles to learn about putting children to sleep, returned to Philadelphia soon after he arrived.[24] Dr. Deming was a pioneer in her own right, administering anesthesia at a time when the precarious airways of newborns were not routinely protected with a breathing tube. The airway was more vulnerable to obstruction from excessive saliva, vomitus, or swelling in the absence of a breathing tube. Deming became a champion of tracheal intubation, inserting a tube into the airway of every newborn for the duration of an operation, even though the equipment to do so was rudimentary.[25]

Koop later described how he and Deming worked together to devise a suitable tube to inflate the lungs of infants and administer anesthesia:

> There was no equipment to be bought; we made our own. The night before surgery we would fashion endotracheal tubes out of red rubber catheters, file the edges with emery boards to prevent injury to the tracheal mucosa, boil them over a bent wire, hoping they would retain some memory of a curve, and then begin to experiment with anesthetic gases as well as preoperative medication.[26]

The lack of the most basic equipment to care for surgical newborns, such as breathing tubes, ventilators, intravenous catheters, and monitors, made it difficult for pediatric surgery to get off the ground.

The fragility of newborns and the paucity of techniques to revive them came to the attention of the nation on August 7, 1963, when

President Kennedy's youngest son, Patrick Bouvier Kennedy, was born five weeks prematurely. Shortly after birth Patrick developed hyaline membrane disease, a lung disease of premature infants in which the air sacs lacked surfactant, a substance that kept them from collapsing. At that time, hyaline membrane disease affected approximately 25,000 babies per year and was the most common cause of death,[27] accounting for up to 10,000 deaths per year.[28]

Doctors in Cape Cod transferred Patrick to Boston Children's Hospital, where he was treated in a hyperbaric chamber, an environment that engulfed the infant in oxygen under pressure, hoping to force it into the lungs. Patrick's twiglike bronchial tubes were swollen from inflammation and thickened with mucus, leaving scant thoroughfare for the passage of oxygen into and out of his lungs. His alveoli were collapsing from a lack of surfactant that his lungs were too immature to produce. With his lungs failing and no means to ventilate him, Patrick was working harder and harder to breathe. Within forty-eight hours of birth, the president's second son died from respiratory failure.

By 1963 open-heart surgery had been performed, kidneys could be transplanted, and James Watson and Francis Crick had unraveled the structure of DNA, but there was still only a primitive understanding of newborn respiratory physiology and no effective means to support newborns in the grip of respiratory failure. Sixteen years after Koop showed up at CHOP to start a pediatric surgery program, the infrastructure to care for a baby like Patrick still did not exist.

An entirely different scenario would unfold for Patrick today. First, if the possibility of a premature birth was suspected, the in utero fetus would be treated with steroids that would accelerate lung maturation prior to delivery. After birth, from the moment Patrick showed any sign of respiratory distress, he would receive synthetic surfactant through a small breathing tube, custom made for babies his size. The tube would be connected to a ventilator to support him until his immature lungs healed. This same technology is used today for babies coming out of anesthesia who are not awake enough to breathe on their own.

Some relief from the hardships of maintaining ivs in pediatric patients finally came in the form of the post–World War II plastics revolution, which brought the ability to make small-caliber tubes with precision.[29] Plastics could be used for almost any type of tube intended for use in the body, from ivs to feeding tubes to urinary catheters and, yes, breathing tubes of all shapes and sizes. Plastics, in a sense, ushered in a golden era of medical devices, and for the first time, single-use devices were available for medical applications.

The first plastic iv catheter that could be inserted through the skin with a needle was conceived in 1950 by Dr. David Massa, an anesthesia resident training at the Mayo Clinic.[30] Tinkering in his basement after hours, Massa soaked a section of pvc tubing in acetone to make it more pliable and threaded it over a steel stylet, or wire, that kept the steel needles from clogging during insertion. He sawed off the hub from a steel needle and attached it to the tubing. He used a cloth buffer to round out the tip of the catheter and then sterilized the entire assembly by heating it in his kitchen oven.

With Massa's catheter-over-needle design, once the sharp tip of the needle was inserted through the skin and penetrated the vein, the pvc catheter was pushed or threaded over the needle into the vein for a distance up to an inch. The needle was then pulled out of the catheter so all that was left in the vein was a pliable, smooth plastic catheter.

When Massa's catheter hit the market in the late 1950s, it sparked an explosion in the development of plastic intravenous catheters. The pvc model was eventually replaced, first by Teflon for its enhanced sliding capability, and later by polyurethane because it was nontoxic. The catheter-over-needle design persists to this day as the predominant configuration of disposable intravenous catheters.[31]

By 1947, pediatric surgeons who had trained in Boston had nested in Philadelphia, Chicago, Seattle, Minneapolis, and Columbus, Ohio. The American Board of Surgery, however, opposed the specialty and refused to acknowledge the special qualifications of pediatric surgeons by granting board certification.

The renegade surgeons were forced to turn elsewhere. They finally found a home, but it was not with fellow surgeons. In 1948, the American Academy of Pediatrics (AAP) admitted twelve surgeons to their organization who were dedicated to the care of children. They called themselves the Surgical Section of the AAP. Affiliating with the nationally known AAP lent the group an air of legitimacy. They could hold annual meetings in conjunction with the AAP annual meeting and became a part of a national platform that addressed and publicized the health priorities of children.[32]

The up-and-coming generation of pediatric surgeons viewed this alignment with pediatricians as a double-edged sword. Dr. Alex Haller at Johns Hopkins described the alliance as an "unnatural marriage" that made it appear that pediatric surgeons were nothing more than operating pediatricians and not "real surgeons" who decided for themselves when to operate and managed their own patients from start to finish.[33]

Whether aligning with the pediatricians was a mistake or not, the perceived taint was finally removed in 1972 with the founding of the independent American Pediatric Surgical Association (APSA), which became the preeminent organization for pediatric surgeons, with members all over the world. Soon after APSA was founded, the American Board of Surgery at last recognized pediatric surgery as a separate subspecialty. For the first time pediatric surgeons would be able to obtain a special certificate of competence in pediatric surgery, the gold standard for any specialty.

Turf battles with general surgeons, other specialists, and pediatricians would continue for decades, but after roughly twenty years of existence, the fledgling specialty at last had a foothold on the territory. Pediatric surgeons could devote their efforts to rescuing children from previously incurable anomalies and diseases and would prove not only that children deserved a higher standard of care than bunny rabbits but also that such a standard was readily achievable.

Half a century after the difficult birth of pediatric surgery, I am able to use a vein that could never have withstood the lacerating bevel of the steel needle ivs of the 1950s. And though even with magnification I can barely see the hole I cut in it, I have tools and techniques refined over fifty years of pediatric surgery practice to assist in the procedure.

I pick up an iris forceps with tips just a half a millimeter wide, the perfect size to grasp the neonatal catheter precisely designed to insert into a tiny premature infant. It has the potential to last for weeks or even months if necessary, an unheard-of expectation for my 1950s predecessors when surgeons were lucky if an iv lasted a few days.

I grasp the catheter as close to the tip as I can and wiggle it into the hole, and once the tip is inside the vein I feed more of the catheter in, one millimeter at a time, while it flops around like an overcooked piece of angel-hair pasta. With a final gentle push, I insert it in all the way to the hub, now six inches in; attach a syringe; pull back gently; and watch as a rush of dark blood flashes into the barrel. This tells me the tip has made it all the way to just inside the right atrium of the heart, the result I was hoping for, one that brings this baby closer to a future.

the shortcut to survival

During an exploratory laparotomy a surgeon cuts through the skin and muscular layers of the abdomen, inspects the organs within, and tries to find a cause for a patient's symptoms. A mix of excitement and anticipation accompanies the beginning rituals of a major operation, as the surgical team squares off the towels around a sterile field, drapes the sheets, wheels the instruments up to the table, and focuses the overhead lights.

Adrenalin runs higher still if the abdomen in question belongs to an infant. With babies, the word "exploratory" is not used lightly. Even with X-rays, ultrasound, and CT scans there is uncertainty, the implicit understanding that in opening up the black box of a human newborn one will possibly catch a glimpse of the infinite nature of variation, of something totally unknown and unexpected, of gestation gone awry.

Will the surgeon find a nameable condition within her power to repair? Or will she encounter something not so easily fixed, a diagnosis that sentences the patient to a series of complicated operations, a situation plagued with setbacks and months of hospitalization? Even worse, will she find organs so grossly malformed or incomplete that she can only palliate and close, becoming the messenger of grief to despairing parents in a darkened hallway? The answer, only minutes away, lurks beneath the skin in the shadow of a scalpel poised and ready.

When surgeons at the Children's Hospital of Philadelphia explored the abdomen of Baby K., a two-day-old infant with persistent vomiting, they were not greeted by the usual loops of small intestine erupting into the operative field like handfuls of slippery balloons. Instead of unruly intestine spilling across the table, her surgeons could find almost none at all.[1] Baby K.'s feedings had come right back up within hours of her swallowing them because there was no place for them to go.

With this malformation, a near total intestinal atresia, the intestine fails to form, likely due to an in utero accident in which it twists into a tight corkscrew, choking off the flow of blood and causing the tissue to die. This type of twisting might affect only a small part of the intestine or its entire length. In Baby K.'s case all that remained after the mishap was an inch or two of functional small intestine and remnants of what might have been — knotted strands of shriveled tubes that would never be adequate to support a life. The year was 1967, and up until that point in history, it was a malformation that no one was expected to survive.

An operating room discovery like this can sneak up on a surgeon. After the buildup, the whisper of the scalpel drawing back the curtain on a mystery, one can almost hear the rush of air as a vacuum threatens to suck every molecule out of the room. A surgeon may have a decade of training, twenty years of experience, and an array of shiny tools second to none, but there's nothing she can do, nothing that will make any measurable difference to the life of this baby. Standing at the table in this moment, the energy level tamps down. The music stops. The joy is gone.

Most of us choose this job of surgeon because we like the quick fix — the opportunity to wave our magic wand, the scalpel, and set a life back on course again. We don't want to spend hours on rounds contemplating obscure medical diseases or staring at bacteria darting in and out of pressed glass bubbles under a microscope. We would rather be getting our hands dirty and using them to save a life than making a living pondering the fate of desperately ill patients from a distance.

But then we encounter an impasse, like this one, that no amount of cleverness will surmount.

When the surgeon regroups after the disappointment and begins mopping up before closing, she might think back to how she explained the operation to the parents in the first place. What exact words did she use? Was it a canned speech or did she improvise? Was she too optimistic? Did she make it sound like everything was going to be okay when really she had no clue? How will she backtrack now from *These things usually go just fine* (which they do) to *I'm afraid I've got some bad news* (that will change your lives forever)?

No surgeon likes the feeling of knowing she can't save a patient's life, but we've all been there too many times. In my first year of practice, I was consulted about a newborn vomiting green with a probable bowel obstruction. Her X-rays showed a dilated loop of intestine and a cutoff in the intestinal gas pattern. The baby had passed hardly any stool. An X-ray of the colon showed that the caliber was small, consistent with a newborn bowel obstruction, probably a blockage somewhere. I drove in to see the baby, and when I pulled back her blanket to examine her, I saw something I'd never seen before—a small black piece of dried-up tissue, hanging to the right of the umbilical cord. It could easily have been mistaken for the umbilical cord, since the two were so similar in appearance, but they were separate structures.

The dried fragment was unusual. I touched it, took a photo. I thought to myself, this almost looks like a miniature replica of the intestine, but no, that's impossible. That doesn't happen. At least I'd never seen a picture in a textbook or heard of such an anomaly. I knew that the intestine exited the abdomen in utero through the umbilicus, ventured out into the amniotic cavity, turned around, and came back in, and the hole closed behind it. I wondered, mainly out of curiosity, without any undue concern, whether this hole could have closed early in gestation. *Could that quarter-sized black thing actually be a shrunken piece of intestine?*

When I opened the baby's abdomen minutes later I fully expected to find a repairable blockage of some kind, but no small intestine bubbled out to greet me. I opened the incision wider and looked around, and there was virtually none. And then the dots instantly connected in my mind like the stars of the Big Dipper imprinted on a stark winter sky—that thing hanging on the outside, the lack of air on X-ray, finding just a couple of inches of small intestine inside my patient.

Now I knew.

The scenario I had considered, but did not know enough to fear, had indeed taken place. My patient had an in utero gastroschisis, an extremely rare condition where the small intestine moved outside the abdomen to rotate, but the hole closed before it could get back inside, cutting off the small intestine's blood flow.

The only thing left to do was to connect the two ends together and close. This was in the early 1990s, twenty years after the birth of Baby K., and still the outlook hadn't changed all that much. One day the future would start to brighten for patients born without enough viable intestine to support their growth and development, but not in time for my young patient. She would never be able to absorb enough nutrition to be a long-term survivor.

The small intestine, that part of the gastrointestinal tract where 95 percent of nutrient absorption takes place, is essential for life. As the roots of a plant draw nutrients from the soil, so does the intestine draw nourishment from ingested food. After the stomach mixes and liquefies what we eat, digestive enzymes and bile secreted by the pancreas and liver are dumped into the slurry as it moves into the duodenum, the first part of the intestine.[2]

As the bolus moves through the gastrointestinal tract, digestion continues—proteins are disassembled into amino acids, fats into fatty acids, and carbohydrates into simple sugars. These elemental nutrients, what will become the future building blocks of all the body's processes, are then absorbed through the intestinal lining, the mucosa, through fingerlike projections, the microvilli. From there the molecules pass into blood vessels in the wall of the intestine and eventually flow via the portal vein to the liver. The material that remains unabsorbed, such as fiber, continues on to the large intestine and is eventually excreted in the stool.[3]

In general, the body harbors an ample supply of small intestine, up to twenty-two feet in an adult and ten feet in a young child. There is so much small intestine, in fact, that a substantial part of it can be removed, up to 60 percent or more, and there will be no noticeable effects. When the intestine is diseased or injured to the extent that a massive loss of length results, however, the body is unable to absorb sufficient nutrients, a condition labeled "short bowel syndrome."

Short bowel syndrome, uncommon but devastating, occurs in 120 of every 100,000 live births. The most common causes in newborns are intestinal atresias, a malformation where some portion of intestine fails to form, similar to Baby K.'s condition. Necrotizing enterocolitis, a disease of premature infants where vast segments of small and large intestine become inflamed and in severe cases must be removed, is the second most common cause. A twisting of the entire small intestine, a midgut volvulus, may occur before or after birth and, if not corrected in time, can destroy most of the small intestine.[4]

Adults can also become victims of short bowel syndrome, although the major causes differ. A motor vehicle accident or gunshot wound can transect the blood vessels that feed the entire intestine. The small intestine can become diseased beyond repair from inflammatory bowel disease or an acute vascular accident involving the main intestinal arteries.

No matter what the cause, when a patient suddenly loses the majority of his intestine he is said to have had an "abdominal catastrophe," as the situation presents an imminent threat to survival.

If these patients are to survive at all, they must rely on some other source of nutrition.

Baby K.'s surgeons sewed the blind-ending first portion of her intestine, the duodenum, to the nubbin of small intestine that connected to her colon. A blockage in her colon was diverted with a colostomy, and a drainage tube, a gastrostomy, was placed into her stomach. As she had virtually no small intestine, feeding her by mouth was not an option because nothing would be absorbed. Instead, doctors kept her on intravenous fluids that contained the maximum concentration of calories that could be given by vein: a 10 percent solution of glucose with added protein and electrolytes. They could not, however, give her enough of the solution to meet all of her caloric needs: there were limits to the amount of fluid they could administer to a five-pound infant without flooding her heart and lungs.

Over the ensuing nineteen days Baby K.'s weight dropped to four pounds from her birth weight of five pounds. Her eyes appeared sunken. Her skin hung loosely from her arms and legs. She became lethargic, her movements slowed by the gradual starvation taking place. She stopped responding to external stimuli. Her doctors had exhausted every medical and surgical option available. There was nothing more they could do to reverse the dismal trend.

In 1967, the idea of infusing high concentrations of nutrients such as glucose, protein, and fat into a patient's veins, enough calories to sustain life indefinitely, was not considered possible, practical, or affordable. The predominant opinion was that postoperative patients could not handle the vast amounts of fluid necessary to convey sufficient calories, that it would tip them into pulmonary edema or even heart failure. Another concern was that the high glucose levels necessary to provide sufficient calories would be dangerous.

The obvious solution was to concentrate the nutrients into smaller volumes so that more calories could be delivered in a smaller volume of fluid. These concentrated nutrient infusions, however, would cause a burning sensation and produce a caustic, chemical irritation to extremity veins. The veins would become inflamed and clotted with stagnant blood and possibly even infected. Furthermore, the overall safety of infusing concentrated nutrients into the body was still unknown, and there were concerns about liver toxicity and the potential for blood infections.

The prevailing practice in the 1960s, therefore, was to use only dilute concentrations of glucose, saline, and electrolytes to supplement patients through short-term illnesses that impaired the function of the gastrointestinal tract. Patients with reversible conditions would hopefully recover with temporary nutritional support. But patients with chronic conditions that extended over months would wither away as their energy reserves were depleted with each passing day. Surgical wounds that required increased calories to heal would break down and fall apart. Immune systems would weaken, and patients would eventually succumb to organ failure or infection.

At the University of Pennsylvania Hospital Dr. Stanley Dudrick, a general surgery resident in 1967, had been deeply affected by the ravages of postoperative malnutrition. When he was an intern in charge of postoperative care, three of his patients died within days of each other.[5] He blamed himself and wondered what he could have done differently to change the outcome.

What had he missed that would have made a difference? Had a deadly infection gone undiagnosed, a correctable electrolyte abnormality? Had he failed to detect a harbinger of disaster on physical exam?

Dudrick's chief of surgery, Dr. Jonathan Rhoads, pointed out that the patients' deaths hadn't been his fault at all. Their recoveries had been complicated by poor nutritional states. All three were saddled with complex gastrointestinal problems that had impaired their ability to eat for weeks to months before undergoing major operations. While the actual operations had gone as well as expected, all patients recovering from abdominal operations experience a period of time when intestinal function ceases. This phenomenon, which can affect patients of all ages, is known as an "ileus" and typically lasts for several days to weeks, a time during which patients cannot tolerate oral feedings. Dudrick's postoperative patients, at a disadvantage from the start, had simply run out of nutritional reserves to fuel their recoveries.

Surgeons have historically been concerned with nutrition for several reasons. First, it was surgeons who usually cared for patients with severe intestinal disorders, many of whom would become malnourished as their conditions worsened. Second, poor nutrition can affect a patient's outcome after a major operation by impairing wound healing, leading to complications and affecting overall morbidity and survival. It was surgical patients — victims of multiple trauma, major burns, inflammatory bowel disease, and cancer, conditions that increase caloric expenditure — who used up their nutritional reserves. Simply undergoing a major abdominal operation and thus being unable to eat for an extended period of time was enough to put a patient into a nutritional hole.

When dietary intake is at normal levels, the body uses glucose as its main energy source. Glucose is obtained from the breakdown of ingested sugars and carbohydrates, but if these are lacking, glucose can be obtained from the breakdown of glycogen (sugar) stores in the liver. At about six hours into fasting, when glycogen stores are starting to run low, the body breaks down stored fat into glycerol and fatty acids and converts them to sources of energy. After several days of continued fasting, the body starts to break down protein from skeletal muscle to meet energy needs.

A similar process unfolds when the body is under major stress, such as trauma, major surgery, or overwhelming infection. It releases hormones that mobilize fat and protein stores, a process known as "catabolism." The body starts to feed on itself, much as it does during fasting, but at an accelerated rate, depleting first fat stores and then muscle. This results in an increased availability of energy substrates such as amino acids that provide proteins to manufacture infection-fighting agents and to provide the building blocks for wound healing. If this process continues unabated, a patient's limited nutritional reserves become depleted over the course of roughly a week and a half.

In the case of a child, the body's nutritional reservoirs are drained even faster. Children have higher baseline energy requirements to begin with, partly due to rapid growth and development. Being smaller, with less muscle mass, they have half the amount of stored protein as adults. Fat stores, which typically increase with age, are particularly limited in newborns.[6] Respiratory distress increases the work of breathing and expends calories. Bloodstream infections and other types of critical illness tax the energy reserves of pediatric patients, especially babies, more than adults. Baby K.'s lack of intestine left her vulnerable to severe malnutrition, and her life was endangered within only weeks.

Dudrick was not the first to experiment with intravenous nutrition, but he had a novel idea about how to get an adequate amount of calories into a patient's bloodstream to ensure survival. He postulated that infusing concentrated nutrient solutions into the larger, central veins of the body, where there was a higher rate of blood flow, would allow the nutrients to be rapidly diluted. Once the nutrients were diluted in the central venous circulation, they would not be as caustic to the veins.

He then developed a technique of threading a longer-than-normal intravenous catheter from a peripheral extremity vein all the way into the superior vena cava at its junction with the right atrium, where there was a much higher rate of blood flow. This development was pivotal because the success of administering the concentrated nutritional solutions depended on reliable access to the larger, core veins in the body. These catheters came to be known as central venous catheters, or central lines, and the technique of infusing nutrients into the central venous system was labeled Total Parenteral Nutrition (TPN).

Dudrick would need to conduct experiments to see, first, whether his technique worked (i.e., could he get an immature animal to grow with TPN?) and, second, whether this method was safe over the long term. Maintaining central lines in active puppies would be challenging, and at that time there were no catheters small and soft enough to insert into a small animal and long enough to thread all the way to the heart. Dudrick made a trip to the local Pep Boys auto parts store, where he purchased a spool of polyvinylchloride (PVC) tubing that was used as insulation for electrical cables. Back at the lab he tested the tubing's heat tolerance to autoclave sterilization and implanted it in animals to see how the body would react.[7]

Ultimately, the setup to infuse the puppies consisted of the PVC tubing that was used as the central venous catheter, speedometer cable (also from Pep Boys) that was used to protect the IV tubing after it exited the puppies' back, and a swivel apparatus (developed by the university's engineering department) that attached to the top of the cage and allowed the dogs to be mobile without pulling out their IVs.

The experiments were labor intensive, and Dudrick had to do everything himself. He mixed the IV solutions. He hung the bags and changed them every day. He weighed the puppies, measured their urine output, and analyzed the chemical composition of the urine to determine the ideal mix of electrolytes and nutritional components.

Using puppies from the same litter, he divided them into two groups; one group was nourished solely with TPN, and the other was fed orally. Within six weeks, the TPN nourished puppies had outstripped the weight gain of their orally fed littermates and suffered no complications. Based on these preliminary results, Dudrick was permitted to treat six hospitalized adult patients, all of whom were severely malnourished after suffering from chronic gastrointestinal problems. Under Dudrick's regimen, all six recovered and were discharged.

Meanwhile, at the children's hospital across town, word of Dudrick's success growing puppies had reached one of Baby K.'s surgeons, the young Dr. Diller Groff, who had interned with Dudrick. By this time, Baby K. was languishing, on a certain path to death. With a sense of urgency Groff phoned Dudrick and asked him to present the results of his experiments the next day at the children's hospital's grand rounds.

Dudrick presented his data to the group. At the end of his talk he was pelted with questions from the crowded auditorium, but the one that stands out in his mind was from his surgical colleague Groff: "Can you play your puppy trick on this baby we have?"[8]

Dudrick agreed to consult on the feasibility of providing nutritional therapy to Baby K.

"She appeared cachectic, hypometabolic and moribund," he later recalled regarding his first impression of Baby K. "It was obvious she was dying of starvation."[9]

He recognized immediately that it would be a monumental undertaking to adapt the nutritional treatment used in the puppies and six adults to a newborn baby, but he also realized that Baby K. was not going to survive otherwise. If Groff could muster support from the staff at the children's hospital, Dudrick would take on the challenge of adapting the technology to treat Baby K.

But there was another substantial hurdle that had to be dealt with first.

No one had ever administered TPN to a baby, and to do so for the first time would require close monitoring for potential complications and attention to every detail to avoid a mishap. If Baby K. suffered a complication or failed to improve, it could be a major setback for the wider acceptance of TPN. A further concern was the ethical consequence of treating Baby K., who most likely did not have sufficient small intestine to sustain long-term survival. Would TPN only prolong what was then viewed as a hopeless condition? At that point no one knew for sure whether or not TPN would allow Baby K.'s intestine to develop sufficiently to support a close to normal life, because this was a treatment that had never been undertaken in a child.

Physicians can be punishing critics when it comes to implementing new medical techniques that disrupt the status quo. Guided by the principle *Primum non nocere*, "First do no harm," they tend to stick with safe, proven methods even when the potential upside to a new treatment is substantial. Dudrick understood this. Appreciating the inherent controversy and risk of the treatment he was about to undertake, he assembled an ad hoc committee to consider not only the medical aspects of Baby K.'s condition but also the ethical questions surrounding treating her. Neonatologists, pediatric surgeons, laypeople, and clergy were involved in the discussions. They met for an entire day in a large auditorium where anyone was welcome to participate and ask questions.

Dudrick explained that they were entering almost entirely uncharted waters. He told the group not to expect success and to be prepared for "potholes" along the way. He made it clear he wouldn't undertake the high-risk therapy without the full support of the team, and they had to be ready to change course if the therapy proved too dangerous or was not effective. In light of Baby K.'s near terminal state, the committee deemed the risks worth even a sliver of potential benefit and endorsed treating Baby K. with TPN.[10]

As Dudrick later readily acknowledged, instituting a relatively untested treatment virtually overnight in a newborn would be next to impossible in today's heavily regulated environment. Dudrick's innovation fortuitously managed to slip in under the wire when it entered the clinical arena, before institutional review boards (IRBs) had become a mainstay in medical research.

Conceived on the heels of what were deemed to be ethical

abuses in medical research that were recognized during and after World War II, IRBs serve as independent ethics committees to review and approve biomedical and other research on human subjects. They regard the safety of human subjects as the top priority in reviewing proposed studies. IRB committees are particularly sensitive to studies involving children, where informed consent must be obtained by proxy — through a parent or legal guardian. Before the advent of IRBs, there was little oversight of medical research.

The Tuskegee Syphilis Study, conducted between 1932 and 1972 by the US Public Health Service in rural Alabama, was a perfect example of how research priorities can become misguided without oversight. The study followed the long-term effects of syphilis in a population of African American males, but the research subjects were never told they had been diagnosed with syphilis and therefore were not afforded the opportunity to be treated and potentially cured of the disease. The National Research Act of 1974 empowered IRBs to review all research that was supported, directly or indirectly, by the Department of Health and Human Services — in effect, all research conducted in medical schools throughout the United States.[11]

After Dudrick's ad hoc committee approved the proposed treatment, Dudrick went back to his laboratory and assembled the equipment he would need to begin TPN infusions in Baby K. He would have to insert a central venous catheter, the first such feat in a baby. He used the same PVC tubing he inserted in the puppies.

To implant the catheter he made a small incision in Baby K.'s neck and inserted a 24-gauge catheter, the width of a broom straw, into a branch of the internal jugular vein and threaded it into her superior vena cava, the largest vein in the body that drained into the heart. He then tunneled the catheter behind her ear, exiting through her scalp, so that she wouldn't inadvertently pull it out when she rolled over in her crib.

He started the TPN infusion with a conservative mixture of hypertonic dextrose, amino acids, and the electrolytes sodium chloride and potassium. Other essential elements were added one by one—calcium, phosphorous, magnesium, and vitamins—so that the medical personnel could note whether any of the additives caused an adverse reaction.[12]

Forty-five days later Baby K.'s weight had almost doubled, she had grown two inches, and her head circumference was approaching normal. Over the ensuing months she was transformed from an emaciated, skeleton of a baby into a chubby-cheeked, active infant of eighteen pounds.[13]

Along the way to this amazing result, numerous clinical hurdles were traversed, most for the first time, and many of which required creative solutions. For example, at the time there was no commercially available source of intravenous fat to provide the essential fatty acids. As a consequence, Baby K. developed flaky dry skin and total body dandruff, signs of essential fatty acid deficiency. Dudrick instructed her parents to eat a high-fat breakfast—eggs, buttered toast, sausage, and whole milk. An hour later he drew a blood sample and spun it down in a centrifuge to isolate the fatty component. He then infused the fatty emulsion from her parents' blood into Baby K. Within a few days, the rash began to clear, and eventually it completely resolved. The infusions continued once a month for the remainder of her treatment with TPN. This allowed Baby K.'s parents to contribute to her care and in this small way to be a part of her.

During the course of Baby K.'s treatment, clinicians and scientists gathered vast quantities of data to use in refining intravenous nutrition for the benefit of future generations of patients, and they willingly shared it with colleagues. The preliminary findings were quickly published so that the word could get out to those who were treating patients in need. When news of Baby K.'s response to therapy spread, Dudrick was contacted by colleagues from Harvard, Yale, and Johns Hopkins, all of whom were anxious to visit Philadelphia, learn the technique, and introduce it as soon as possible at their home institutions.

Numerous other inventions and ideas sprung out of Baby K.'s treatment, including the importance of administering intravenous vitamin D to prevent rickets (as well as how much to give), the development of Betadine ointment to coat the skin around the exit site of a central venous catheter to prevent infections, the use of a final filter between the IV tubing and the patient to increase the sterility of the intravenous solutions, and the development of an intravenous form of a multivitamin solution rather than intramuscular injections.

Dudrick was dogged in his pursuit of finding solutions to the many clinical conundrums that arose during Baby K.'s treatment. He devised workarounds for products he needed and found ways to plead his case to the higher-ups in pharmaceutical and medical device companies so they would manufacture those products. He knew that the success of the mission rested with addressing each and every detail, and once he had identified a need for a new product, he would not accept no for an answer.

Sadly, TPN could not extend Baby K.'s life indefinitely. After repeated attempts to transition to oral feedings failed, she ultimately succumbed to a combination of organ failure and infection at twenty-two months of age.

Not everyone agreed with the decision to put Baby K. on TPN because she had a very short length of functional intestine and her chances for full recovery were not good. The introduction of TPN into the therapeutic armamentarium, in fact, raised new controversies for pediatric surgeons and neonatologists alike. Physicians were suddenly empowered with a life-prolonging and, in some cases, lifesaving option for babies who were previously unsalvageable by virtue of the fact that they were intestinal cripples or could not eat and digest food normally for a host of reasons.

What if some patients never recovered enough to be weaned from TPN? Who would decide when the treatment had gone on long enough? Who would pull the plug? With the success of Baby K.'s treatment, pediatric surgeons had no choice but to wade into the murky waters of using artificial means to support patients. TPN had the unintended consequences of blurring the boundaries of what defined ethical treatment.

Small intestine transplant was still decades away. Would some patients become permanent residents of the hospital until they simply ran out of venous access sites or developed another fatal complication such as liver failure or sepsis? What would it cost to maintain an infant in the hospital on TPN indefinitely? How long could a baby, or an adult for that matter, survive on TPN?

In 1967, no one knew the answers to these questions. Dudrick and those who worked with him to treat Baby K. were, in a sense, stumbling in the dark, barely sure of the methods and not at all certain of the long-term consequences; but the potential of this new therapy was huge, and there was no holding it back.

Today TPN is available in virtually every hospital in America, and it has saved countless patients. Over the ensuing five decades, TPN became a self-described "career-long obsession" for Dudrick.[14] He went on to become an accomplished professor, a chairman of surgery, and the guru of intravenous nutrition as he continued to champion the cause of intravenous nutrition worldwide. Fifty years after treating Baby K., however, his reverence for her contribution had not faded.

"We probably learned ninety-five percent of what we know about infant nutrition from that one baby," he later noted.[15] "Her legacy to the clinical application and development of parenteral nutrition is unparalleled."[16]

In today's world, the proposal to treat Baby K. with the relatively untested TPN might not have withstood the scrutiny of a stringent IRB review. Even if it had, hospital lawyers, fearing litigation over an adverse outcome, might have nixed the trial before it ever got started. And today an ethics committee might have excluded Baby K. from consideration based on the fact that TPN was not going to cure her.

In 1967, however, those obstacles did not exist. It was in that narrow window of medical history that the fates of a desperate baby and an innovative surgeon were joined. Through this chance encounter TPN became a reality for infants on the brink of malnutrition and death, a shortcut to survival made possible by the brief life of Baby K.

4

inside out

Only moments had passed since she was pulled out, smeared with blood and dripping amniotic fluid, from a six-inch incision in her mother's uterus. Slippery loops of intestine hung free from her tiny belly like a tangle of garden hose, having escaped her body through a hole in her abdominal wall.

Baby A.'s intestines had lost their way.

Instead of leaving her abdomen, rotating, and reentering as programmed in the first trimester of pregnancy, they had stalled in transit, like an astronaut locked out of the space station with no way back inside. For the duration of the pregnancy they floated outside the body in the amniotic fluid of the uterus, displaced and unfettered—twisting and turning into an unwieldy snarl.

Unlike congenital anomalies that are discreetly concealed beneath the skin, Baby A.'s was unavoidably on display. A crowd gathered when she was first brought into the NICU—doctors, nurses, and students. They leaned in to see what this thing, a gastroschisis, would look like. Yes, they had skimmed photos in textbooks, watched PowerPoints at medical conferences, and maybe even seen the healed scar of a baby in some phase of recovery, but to be at the bedside at this moment was like having a front-row seat to a movie about earthquakes in an IMAX theater. The view was both horrifying and fascinating.

As I unwrapped the temporary dressing, a sticky saline-soaked gauze applied at delivery, I exposed the mound of small intestine

—fused, folded, and congealed into bizarre contours—so many loops that they spilled out of my outstretched hands and onto the bed. I pointed to the wormlike appendix attached to the cecum, the first segment of the colon, and from there traced the remaining curve of the large intestine.

The nurse inserted a tube into the baby's mouth and threaded it through the esophagus and into the air-filled bubble of the stomach poking out of the left side of the abdomen. We watched as the tube went down, indenting and deflating the soft pouch as thick green sludge was evacuated. I reached down to a pea-sized ovary peeking up out of the pelvis and tucked it back inside. Then I slipped my finger a half inch across and palpated the bladder.

The instigator of this grand medical curiosity was a simple hole in the abdominal wall to the right of the umbilicus, the size of a fifty-cent piece. I measured it and palpated the tightness of the ringlike opening on the stalk of the bowel, considering all the findings as I planned my next move.

Babies are amazing creatures. If an adult's intestines were spilling out of his abdomen, he would be in unbearable pain, gasping for air, in need of immediate lifesaving surgery. This baby, however, fresh from labor and delivery, occasionally squirmed and kicked up at my hands but was otherwise in no noticeable distress. We were poking her and shining lights in her eyes, but her intestines had been outside of her body for most of her in utero life; she had lived this way inside her mother for months.

A gastroschisis like Baby A.'s is one of the two major types of abdominal wall defects, occurring in one in every 2,500 live births. The other major type is an omphalocele, similar but with a larger opening in the abdominal wall. More abdominal organs are usually protruding outside the body, and they are covered with a translucent saclike membrane, similar to the lining of the abdomen that covers and encloses the organs. Omphaloceles are generally the more serious of the two types, not only because the

defect is usually larger, potentially taking months longer to resolve, but also because there is a 20 percent incidence of associated malformations, such as a life-threatening heart defect or a
chromosomal anomaly.

Embryology provides the key to understanding how abdominal
wall defects happen in the first place. During gestation the rapidly
growing intestine outstrips its domicile and pushes through the
umbilicus, where it continues to grow and rotate. This happens
with all babies. By the tenth week of gestation the intestine re-
turns to the abdominal cavity, where it forms attachments in the
normal orientation, with the colon curving around the centrally
positioned small intestine.

With abdominal wall defects, however, when the intestine fails
to return, the relatively empty abdominal cavity has no impetus
to enlarge to a size sufficient to accommodate the exiled organs.
While the exact cause for the defect is unknown, one possible explanation is that several intersecting parts of the abdominal wall
musculature fail to completely fuse, thereby leaving behind a gap
that becomes the hole in the abdominal wall.

My bond with Baby A. had begun weeks earlier, when I first met
with her parents-to-be in my office to discuss the unexpected abnormality detected during a routine prenatal ultrasound. The obstetrician had found dilated loops of intestine extending outside
the abdominal wall early in gestation, around eighteen weeks, an
almost certain sign of gastroschisis.

The young couple huddled in my office were expecting their
first child. They held hands as I showed them color photographs
from *The Atlas of Pediatric Surgery*, pointing out the difference between an omphalocele, a dome-shaped purplish mass protruding
like the head of an eggplant, and a gastroschisis, where the intestines hang free and exposed. In the orchestrated chaos of gestation almost any imaginable defect might emerge, but when the
abdomen split apart, causing internal organs to protrude as if a

baby had been turned inside out, the sight was alarming and easily terrified young parents.

Their eyes widened as I showed them how their baby would look when she first came out: loops of intestine would be draped across the abdomen like pink and purple sausages shot through with a bright red net of blood vessels. The sight was so disturbing that eighteenth-century physicians, perplexed as to how or why the abnormality could possibly have occurred, deemed afflicted infants "monsters."[1]

Grasping for an explanation, physicians theorized that midwives had manhandled the baby during delivery, exerted too much pressure on the baby's abdomen, and thereby caused it to rupture.[2] These babies, healthy in all respects except for the displacement of their intestines, would be deemed unsalvageable and left to die until the dawn of the 1900s. Once antibiotics were available the babies were guarded from infection when the intestines were placed back inside, and their survival considerably improved.

All parents are fearful when meeting for the first time with a pediatric surgeon, by definition someone trained to cut their baby open on the first day of life and rearrange her organs. They can hardly conceive of a newborn requiring an emergency operation, much less the complex anatomical variants that prompt the need. While this is a routine anomaly to pediatric surgeons, one of the more common ones we deal with in the neonatal intensive care unit, the concept scares parents and anyone else who has never seen or heard of a gastroschisis.

We reviewed the stages of repair and how the abdomen would look when the organs were back inside. All that would be left was a simple, nonthreatening hole, so small that one could imagine it could be closed almost effortlessly. We ended on the final pictures —a barely noticeable suture line, a resolving scar, a baby who looked like a completely intact infant.

Their faces started to soften as the thought swept through

their minds. *As bad as it sounds, "the guts on the outside of the body," this could turn out okay.* This was one of the best parts of the job, providing comfort to anxious parents before you even met your patient-to-be, trying to reassure them that there was a way out of this scary scenario that would provide a normal life for their child.

We couldn't know for sure how it would all turn out, but of all the abnormalities to be born with, a gastroschisis was one of the better ones if there were no complications. It was a big "if" that we surgeons lived with every day. We didn't have a crystal ball and could not be sure that we would be mistake-free every single outing or that the patient wouldn't throw us a curve ball with a variant of anatomy or some other unexpected vulnerability. We reminded the family and ourselves that everything *could* turn out okay, knowing better than to ever use the word "will."

What if you can't get it all back in? It was an obvious question and one that parents predictably asked with worry etched on their faces.

I thought back to the early years of my career, when getting the organs back in as quickly as possible on the first day of life was the main goal. Every patient was taken to the operating room and put under general anesthesia, an ordeal accompanied by hours of preparing for the operation placing intravenous lines for fluid infusion and monitoring. When it came time to prep, we would pour Betadine across the intestines, lift them up with gloved hands, and place sterile towels and drapes around the hole in the abdomen. We would hover over the baby in a sweltering operating room, inspecting the pile of swollen, matted intestine, wondering not whether we could get it all back in but what it would take to do so.

We would incise the skin to open up the hole if necessary so we would have more room to work. If a loop curved to the right, we would push it in and angle it close to the liver. The next one veering toward the right or left would snug in under the ribs on that side, below the stomach on the left or the liver on the right. While some loops would tuck into the upper quadrants, others would fold down into the lower pelvis. Sometimes the entire intestine could be inserted into the abdomen with relatively little effort. Other times the compartment was too small, and getting the intestines back in was like trying to force a size 9 foot into a size 7 shoe. We would take curved metal retractors, hook them into the abdominal wall, and pull it as far apart as possible so we could force more loops inside. With luck and persistence we would be able to shoehorn everything back in, not necessarily a comfortable fit but one that achieved the desired result of primary closure.

When the intestine didn't all fit back in, we would have to pull the loops back out, cover them with warm moist sponges, and start over. Then we would insert gloved fingers inside the undersized abdominal cavity, two on one side, two on the other, and pull from top to bottom, gently stretching the muscles and skin, trying to make a little more room, enough to get that last loop back inside.

The part of me that had been there many times before knew that with patience these various maneuvers, in concert, were probably going to work. But there was also a sliver of doubt, that tiny voice I nearly always kept muzzled, if not entirely crated, in the back of my mind, the voice that stands with arms folded, foot tapping, shaking its head while staring at the clock, chiding me for taking too long, undermining my confidence.

But I would just keep working, tucking one loop at a time back inside, ignoring the color, the loops turning from pink to pale to gray as the blood vessels that fed the intestine were subtly compromised, noting the ventilator pressures as they steadily climbed. *Give more paralytics. Turn up the anesthesia. Get me some room to work in there*, I would implore the anesthesiologist. The rising intra-abdominal pressure would squeeze off the blood flow to the kidneys, causing the urine output to drop to near zero for days.

My surgical training, like that of my colleagues, was inscribed on my frontal cortex and held the same weight as the tablets handed down from Moses. The directive was simple and clear. *Do everything you can to get the organs back in.* And for every single case, I dutifully donned the blinders and did my best to do so.

But there were a few times when everything would not fit back in no matter what we did. The maneuvers failed, the anatomy betrayed us, and we simply had to concede. We would have to go to Plan B.

There wasn't much deliberation or doubt, because we had tried every possible way to get the intestine back in and it just wasn't going to happen on that particular day. By then we had maxed out the sedatives and paralytics. The intestines, swollen and taut with fluid, were starting to split apart like overripe peaches and threatening to rupture. The baby was packed so tightly that the diaphragms could barely move, the lungs couldn't expand, and the oxygen saturations would plunge. There wasn't going to be any more pushing or packing of any kind without killing the baby. But then what would we do next? We couldn't just leave the guts hanging exposed outside the body. We had to find something to cover them to keep them from drying out and shriveling up.

And now we had reached the point in an operation that would test a surgeon's mettle. Could she think outside the box, improvise a solution, stay calm while she looked around the operating room for some way to fabricate a covering? In the early 1990s there wasn't anything commercially available to cover the intestines and seal the hole, so you had to make your own. What was needed was a vertical cylindrical structure patterned after a grain silo except, instead of holding wheat or corn, it could hold intestines. The surgeon would have to sew one end of the silo around the hole where the intestines came out of the body and tie off the other end to keep them from escaping. In this way the intestines could be suspended upright, outside and on top of the abdomen; gravity would gradually pull them back into the abdomen while the incoming contents slowly stretched the interior cavity.

Dr. Sam Schuster was one of the first to create an improvised silo to treat a large omphalocele in 1959.[3] He sutured a small sheet of Teflon mesh to the edges of the abdominal muscle on each side of the hole in the abdominal wall, pulled the pieces snug, and sutured them together. Then he closed the baby's skin over the mesh. Each week he would take the patient to the operating room, open the skin, snug the mesh down some more, and excise the excess material as the abdominal cavity slowly enlarged and the muscles stretched to accommodate the intestine. Eventually the mesh could be removed entirely, and the two edges of the abdominal musculature and the skin could be brought together and closed.

Eventually this technique evolved into sewing a Silastic sheet, a sterile flexible plastic wrapping, circumferentially around the abdominal defect, to the full thickness of the abdominal wall, the edges of the Silastic sewn together along the side and over the top in a chimney configuration. Some sort of antibiotic-impregnated dressing was then placed over this external covering. Each day, the chimney was cinched up and made smaller by pushing the intestine down as far as it would easily go and applying a tie around the end of the Silastic chimney. Variations of the chimney would continue to evolve over the ensuing decades.[4]

The materials available for a surgeon to use might depend on where she was working: whether the hospital was well equipped, like a state-of-the-art children's hospital, or whether she was at the county hospital, where only the most rudimentary equipment was available and nothing was stocked for babies. Some surgeons emptied iv bags and hastily sewed them together in the operating room like frantic dressmakers on opening night with the curtain about to go up. The lucky ones were provided sterile sheets of Silastic, or if the defect was smaller they could use a square of Gore-Tex that could be cut to fit around the hole. Desperate surgeons had even packed the intestines into a surgical glove, sewn the base to the hole, and twisted the fingers up with a tie.

No matter what was used, these constructed-on-the-fly coverings had their shortcomings. Abdominal fluid leaked out in between sutures, causing dehydration and increasing the baby's intravenous fluid needs. It was difficult to keep the abdomen and its contents clean, thereby increasing the risk of infection. The covers could be cumbersome to work with, because what was needed was something that could be rolled down a little bit every day, like squeezing a tube of toothpaste, to help reduce the contents back into the abdomen. There was no good way to squeeze the patched-together versions down to force the contents back into the abdomen. Surgeons also worried that the excessive handling required to change the improvised coverings would injure the intestine, especially if it got stuck to the sides of the material.

All of this added up to the working philosophy that, rather than dealing with the hassle of improvising a temporary covering, the method of choice was to force the intestine back in as quickly as possible, usually on the first day of life.

Baby A.'s entire small intestine and most of her colon is hanging outside her undersized abdominal cavity, one that failed to expand to normal size without the pressure of the intestine pushing it from the inside. Her organs have lost their intended domain and will need to be housed in a safe comfortable covering until they can be easily inserted back inside. But I won't have to play dressmaker and improvise with overlapping sheets of plastic that are cumbersome to deal with, because today we have a medical device that was manufactured for the exact purpose of containing the intestine outside the body.

Many pediatric surgeons practicing today have never heard of Dr. James Fischer. His name isn't on the cover of any major textbooks, and he isn't on the faculty of a marquee medical school, but without Fischer, the device that changed the entire management of gastroschisis might not exist.

In the late 1980s, after spending his first sixteen years in practice at the University of Alberta in Edmonton, Alberta, Fischer, a Canadian by birth, moved to Loma Linda University in California. He was only there for two years, but during that time he became familiar with a small medical device company, Bentec Medical, a company that supplied some other items Fischer had used on patients.

Fischer had been sewing in a thick Silastic mesh when he couldn't get a gastroschisis defect closed on the baby's first day of life. Because the Silastic was thick, it was stiff and difficult to manage. There was no ideal way to secure the mesh in position and attach it to the abdominal wall. The mesh was sutured in place with a long continuous suture that went all the way around the hole. All of these difficulties added up to an increased risk of infection, and because the mesh was so thick, Fischer couldn't see through it. He couldn't inspect the color and contour of the bowel, so if there were a problem developing on the inside the covering, he wouldn't be able to see it beneath the covering.

To complicate matters further, the incidence of gastroschisis in Fischer's practice was starting to increase—a trend that continues today. No one is certain why, but environmental toxins and prenatal substance abuse have been cited as possible causes.

"I felt there had to be a way to manage these infants in a quicker, safer manner," he later said.[5]

He conferred with a salesman from Bentec, a company that had both engineering and manufacturing capabilities, and laid out some simple specifications. Fischer needed a bag that could be easily inserted and removed, one in the shape of a flexible preformed silo. The bag would need to be made of a pliable material so it would easily slide over the intestines and could be handled and rolled down easily as the bowel was reduced back into the abdomen. Ideally the bag would be transparent so that the viability of the intestines could be monitored just by looking through it.

While the prevailing view at the time was that it was best to take the infant to the operating room and reduce the extruded organs back into the abdomen as quickly as possible, new information about the consequences of doing so was starting to emerge.

In the early 1990s, abdominal compartment syndrome, a menacing rise in abdominal pressure that can damage intra-abdominal organs and cause respiratory distress, was beginning to be recognized as a cause of complications and mortality in adult trauma patients. Researchers found that even a modest increase in intra-abdominal pressure could decrease the blood flow to internal organs and have a lasting effect on function. This new information raised concerns about forcing organs back into babies with gastroschisis and omphalocele too quickly and paved the way for a staged approach where the contents were worked back in gradually.

Nine months after Fischer's request Bentec produced the first preformed silo bags. The first time he saw them, he knew they were a "great innovation." The Bentec spring-loaded silo bag (sls) was a bag that fit Fischer's specifications perfectly and then some. What distinguished the Bentec bag from anything that had previously been conceived was a collapsible stainless steel ring made up of coils like a Slinky attached to the base of the bag and covered with Silastic. After measuring the defect and choosing the appropriate size, the surgeon slid the sls over the intestine like a sleeve. He then simply pinched the collapsible springlike base of the bag together, like pinching a rubber band into the shape of a hairpin, and inserted it through the hole in the abdomen, where it would resume its previous round shape. When the bag was pulled up taut, the spring held it snug against the front of the abdominal wall. Suturing the bag in place, with its attendant complications, was no longer necessary.

The sls was the first bag that could be placed at the bedside in the nicu with only minimal, if any, sedation of the newborn. Bentec had also included a preformed ring at the end of the bag that was used to suspend it from the top of the isolette (an enclosed crib), thereby enabling gravity to help pull the abdominal contents back inside. Each day the surgeon would go by, squeeze down more of the intestines back into the abdomen, and place a tie around the bag just above where the intestines were situated.

The Bentec SLS was less a technological marvel than a genius of design packaged in simplicity. As simple as it was, however, the new bag fueled a great leap in the treatment of gastroschisis. There were the obvious benefits of avoiding a trip to the operating room on the first day of life and the associated trials of general anesthesia, hypothermia, and blood loss. But possibly the biggest contribution of the Bentec bag was the discovery with its widespread and increasing use that babies did better when they didn't have their ex-patriate guts forcibly shoved back into their abdomens on day one of life. Advantages included better long-term function and fewer immediate complications related to inflammatory episodes with the intestine. There was no need to crank up the ventilator because the belly was too tight and the lungs couldn't expand. Many patients needed no ventilation at all.

After only a few years a consensus emerged: newborns were better off with the Bentec bag. Many pediatric surgeons adopted it as the frontline therapy for the treatment of gastroschisis, and the procedure was frequently performed at the bedside with only minimal, if any, sedation. After a few days, when the intestines had settled gradually into the abdomen, the infant was taken to the operating room to have the bag removed and the abdomen closed.

While the advent of the silo improved the babies' outcomes, it did not prevent every complication. Some babies developed complications from the use of the wrong size bag, one that was too tight around the intestine. The intestine could twist or kink in the bag, damaging it further. Up to 15 percent of babies with gastroschisis are born with an atresia, an intestinal blockage caused by a failure of the intestine to form normally. This complication would most likely require a bowel resection and possibly even a colostomy. Even a baby with an uncomplicated gastroschisis could develop a bowel obstruction later in life from kinking or scarring and require another operation to straighten out the intestine. And there was always the possibility of a severe infection developing, either in the abdomen or in the bloodstream.

Bentec took a financial risk and a leap of faith in producing the bag. There were no exhaustive studies to prove the efficacy of the product before the company moved ahead with marketing it. The company had no idea whether Fischer's concept would catch on across the country, whether surgeons would adopt this method of repair and, if so, how rapidly its use would spread. They waded in gently, producing only two sizes of bags. Today seven sizes are available. The Bentec bag was adopted by every major medical center in the United States and in many countries around the world. Hundreds of thousands have been sold.

The privately held Bentec Medical Company is still in business. In fact, it has expanded into products for cardiology, oncology, urology, and many other fields and applications. It is not a huge company like Johnson and Johnson, but it fills the smaller niche markets that require specialized devices.

Shortly after Baby A. arrived in the NICU, I gathered up several feet of coils, the entire length of gut, and slid them into a tapered Bentec silo bag that enveloped the intestine like a sausage casing. The intestines would stay there until they gradually fell back into the abdomen, a combination of gravity and manual pressure gently coaxing them back in over several days. Later, when all the loops were back inside, we would take Baby A. to the operating room, pull her muscles together, suture them closed, and perform a cosmetic closure of the skin.

Late in the evening, the nurses called me just as I was about to walk out the door. *We think the intestine looks a little blue.* Blue is not a good color for the intestine, ever. I turned around walked back down the hallway and took an elevator up to the NICU. Through the bag the intestine looked a little gray, definitely not as pink as earlier, but when I shined my flashlight I could see the etchings of pink pulsating blood vessels. The intestine was alive.

But alive or not, was the intestine in trouble? Was the blood supply to the intestine significantly compromised, or was there some other explanation for this odd color, such as dehydration or simply poor drainage of venous blood out of the silo?

There were other more serious problems that could be causing the ominous color — there could be a kink in the blood supply to the intestine, choking off the blood flow, or a clot in the superior mesenteric artery that fed the entire small intestine; the intestine could be twisted on itself, or there could be too much pressure in the bag from being packed too tightly.

The color concerned me, but the baby's heart rate was high and the urine output was minimal. I decided Baby A. was probably dehydrated, and I asked the nurses to give a fluid bolus and turn up the iv fluids.

But once I got home, I couldn't help thinking about the color of that intestine. I had seen absolute disasters with silos. I had walked up to the bedside to inspect the silo before only to find that a damaged piece of intestine had blown out, leaving a thick paste of stool smudging the once clear, see-through bag. I had seen a segment turn black after twisting because the blood supply was kinked off and the intestine was dead. As long as the intestine was in the bag, it was vulnerable to technical complications. Being back in the abdomen would not prevent complications, but it would eliminate those associated with the bag.

I remembered how I had reassured the parents that day in my office. My words echoed back to me: *of all the defects to be born with, gastroschisis is one of the better ones.*

I wondered now if I had misspoken. Had it been a mistake to intentionally choose words loaded with hope and favorable expectations, words that I might have to eat now if the intestine became compromised? I knew there was still a long way to go, a path littered with hazards. What if we had to take the bag off and enlarge the hole? They would see it as a setback. What if there was a blockage in the intestine that would have to be repaired weeks from now? Baby A. would be in the hospital for months.

I was reminded yet again that along with my certificate in pediatric surgery, I was not issued a crystal ball. I couldn't predict the outcome any more than I could the weather. All I could do was describe a typical but not guaranteed course, knowing that every patient was different and that in each case all we could do was continue down the road, reading the signs along the way.

Late that night I drove back to the hospital to examine Baby A. again. I could see through the Bentec bag that the color of the intestines had improved. Her vital signs and labs were normal. She was sedated and stable and looked totally normal except for the mass of intestine piled on top of her abdomen.

A few days later I took Baby A. back to the operating room. By that time I had managed to get most of the intestine back inside. When I took the bag off, the intestine pinked up right away and I easily pushed it all back inside the abdomen.

The bag had worked just like Fischer had intended it to, allowing the abdomen to expand just enough so that we could work all the contents back in without stressing Baby A.'s tiny body. A few weeks later she was headed home just like any other healthy baby, with barely a trace of a scar. There were flowers, balloons, and tearful goodbyes to the doctors and nurses who had transformed Baby A. from a baby born inside out to one with a normal life restored and stretched out ahead like an open road.

Because of the Bentec bag, gastroschisis had morphed from an anomaly that was prone to complications to one in which most patients would recover with good outcomes. And all it had taken was a surgeon's ingenuity combined with modern medical device design and materials — an early example of how technology could reshape the entire landscape of a diagnosis. Ahead there were even more amazing, even unthinkable, technologies that would further revolutionize the care of children.

going to extremes

5

Baby X.'s honeymoon is about to end, sooner than expected.

We crowd the blood gas analyzer, watching as it spits out white snippets of paper stippled with fateful numbers. His oxygen level is drifting lower, from mere sag to full-on collapse, while the carbon dioxide climbs like the Dow before the crash.

There are some reassuring signs. He still has a heartbeat. His blood pressure is holding. Heavily sedated, wearing eye patches to block out ambient light, Baby X.'s chest accordions back and forth, the rhythmic blast of the ventilator flexing his sparrow ribs. But what becomes increasingly obvious with each waning report is that the ventilator, now fully maxed out, is not going to be enough. Baby X.'s color has faded from pink to gray. Life is seeping out of him, and soon there will be no more.

How much is left?

Will our next move rally him to survival?

We don't know, but there is only one thing left to try—the most invasive, high-risk therapy that modern technology can muster. What we do next will either save him or prod him to a certain death.

Baby X. is going on ECMO.

Shortly after birth, when Baby X. first had difficulty breathing, his chest X-ray showed what looked like a mass of air bubbles in his left chest. His intestines had slipped up inside his chest, creating multiple air pockets we could see on X-ray. This simple but classic finding tipped his doctors off to the diagnosis of a diaphragmatic hernia — a hole in the diaphragm.

The diaphragm is the dome-shaped muscular shield that separates the abdomen from the chest and aids in respiration, allowing a person to take a deep breath and expand the rib cage. Normally the diaphragm is formed by the fusion of several membranes by the seventh week of gestation. If the diaphragm fails to completely form, leaving a hole between the chest and abdomen, the abdominal contents — the small and large intestine, spleen, stomach, and liver — can slip up into the chest cavity, where they will stay for the remainder of gestation. Consequently, the developing lung bud on the affected side will be compressed. Instead of the lung fully branching out, filling the chest with a spray of spongy pink air sacs, only an underdeveloped bonsai stub of a lung will be present at birth.

When Baby X.'s pediatric surgeon at a nearby hospital operated on him shortly after birth, he found a hole so big that the edges of the diaphragm could not simply be sewn together. He trimmed a patch of Gore-Tex fabric to fit in the shape of the missing muscle and sewed it in place around the circumference of the hole, anchoring it to the ribs along the back edge of the baby's chest because there was only a sparse rim of muscle. The operation was not particularly long or complicated, but no matter how well the pediatric surgeon had done his job, Baby X. still had only a 40 percent chance of surviving because of the underdeveloped lung.

The stable interval between an operation to repair a newborn's diaphragmatic hernia and the almost certain nosedive that follows is referred to as "the honeymoon." No one knows how long the reprieve will last.

Even with the intestines placed back in the abdomen, Baby X. was still susceptible to respiratory failure from pulmonary hypoplasia, or not having enough lung tissue at birth. Adults could live with only one lung, but a baby might not survive with his one normal-size lung plus an underdeveloped piece on the opposite side for two reasons. Not only was the amount of lung tissue deficient for gas exchange (oxygen for carbon dioxide), but also the amount of blood intended to flow through two full lungs would flood the smaller, underdeveloped lung, causing the blood vessels to the lungs to reflexively constrict in both lungs.

This phenomenon, known as pulmonary hypertension, could be unpredictable and overwhelming, more difficult to manage than a ten-foot storm surge after a hurricane, and just as deadly. Bright light, loud noise, too much fluid, too little fluid, touching, jostling, pain—any number of factors could cause the pulmonary arteries to squeeze, choking off the flow of blood trying to get back to the lungs and leaving the rest of the body thirsting for oxygen. Even when the baby was kept perfectly still and sedated in a pitch-black room, the pulmonary hypertension could worsen as the pulmonary arteries pinched down.

Baby X.'s oxygen saturations started to plunge within hours of the operation, leaving his doctors no option but to keep turning up the ventilator settings—adding more oxygen (toxic to a newborn's retinas) and higher pressure (which beat up the lungs). But when Baby X. continued to deteriorate, he was flown by helicopter to the children's hospital, where we had recently started an ECMO (Extracorporeal Membrane Oxygenation) program. When he arrived he was on maximum support, with the ventilator cranked up to the highest settings and intravenous drugs to support his blood pressure, but he was still just barely hanging on.

At the very beginning—in 1965, when Dr. Bob Bartlett dared to think out loud and pose the question during his training at Boston Children's Hospital—ECMO had been an impossible notion.

"Could we use the heart-lung machine to treat acute respiratory failure?" he asked Dr. Robert Gross, the chief of pediatric surgery at Boston Children's, widely regarded as the father of pediatric surgery.[1]

In his usual direct manner, Gross didn't hesitate to inform Bartlett that the machine, as it was then configured in the 1960s, wouldn't work, and why. The heart-lung machine, used to bypass the heart during cardiac surgery, pumped blood out of the body, passed it through an oxygenator that added oxygen and removed carbon dioxide, and pumped it back into the body. But it was designed only for short-term use during open-heart operations. After several hours of churning the blood through the bubble oxygenator, where blood and air came into direct contact, the proteins, red blood cells, and platelets started to get frayed by the friction created between the blood-oxygen interface. Because of this, patients couldn't survive a pump run that extended over several days, the minimum amount of time necessary for the lungs to recover after respiratory failure.

But Bartlett, like most physician inventors, wasn't idly contemplating a fantasy scenario when he first asked the question in 1965. He had just spent two days hand-inflating the lungs of a newborn with a diaphragmatic hernia who had been operated on at birth. The operation had gone well but, after a stable forty-eight-hour "honeymoon," the baby had crashed and died, and there was nothing within medicine's reach that could have prevented it.

Whether a patient's demise is predictable, expected, or unavoidable, losing a patient is personal to a surgeon. He has reached inside his patient's body, manipulated those human organs, and made changes that last a lifetime. Surgeon and patient are forever linked by the outcome of such an intimate endeavor: both of them must live with the consequences. Watching the baby get sucked down the drain of irreversible respiratory failure inspired Bartlett not only to ask the question but also to devote the greater part of his career to answering it.

Bartlett's patient-driven inspiration mirrored that of the surgeon who developed the first successful heart-lung machine, Dr. John H. Gibbon. In 1930 he was working as a research assistant to chest surgeon Dr. Edward Churchill at Massachusetts General Hospital. Churchill was asked to consult on a middle-aged female who was struggling to breathe after gallbladder removal. The presumptive diagnosis was massive pulmonary embolism—a massive blood clot blocking the flow of blood into the patient's lungs and depriving her body of oxygen. Gibbon, the junior member of the team, was instructed to stay at the patient's bedside overnight, record her vital signs every fifteen minutes, and notify the surgical team if she took a turn for the worse.[2]

Gibbons sat at the woman's bedside watching as her neck veins became engorged and her face increasingly dusky as the hours passed and her oxygen level dropped. There was nothing he could do for her other than record her vital signs. He wished for an apparatus that could remove the unoxygenated blood from her veins, infuse it with oxygen, and return it to her body through her arteries.

But there was no such machine in existence.

He watched helplessly as the patient's condition continued to decline. The next morning Churchill took her to the operating room, where he opened her chest and extracted the embolus, but the patient never regained consciousness. This devastating outcome was all the inspiration that Gibbon would need to devote the next nineteen years to developing a heart-lung bypass machine.[3]

Heart surgery was just coming into existence in the 1940s, when Gibbon was completing his training. A smattering of surgeons had started to repair congenital abnormalities in children, such as atrial septal defects ("holes" in the heart) and other life-threatening anomalies. Progress, however, was thwarted by the fact that when surgeons opened the heart, their view of the surgical field was obscured by blood as the beating heart constantly refilled. They were forced to discern the anatomy of the heart by feel and to place sutures into a moving target they could not see. If heart surgery were to advance so that more complex operations could be performed, the heart would need to be still and the surgical field bloodless so that the repair could be performed with precision.

A heart-lung machine would require at least three components: anticoagulation of the blood so that it would not clot when it was routed outside the body, a pump that would replicate the action of the beating heart and move blood back into the body, and an oxygenator, a device to simulate the function of the lungs to infuse venous blood with oxygen while it simultaneously removed carbon dioxide.

While calibrating the degree of anticoagulation would prove to be tricky, heparin had already been discovered and was readily available. There were a variety of industrial pumps, including some from the dairy or food industries, which could be adapted for the heart-lung machine. The more difficult challenge would prove to be the development of an oxygenator, a device that would simulate lung function while the patient was on bypass.

Adult human lungs measure ten to fourteen inches in height and four to six inches across, about the size of a baseball glove. Within the two spongy masses are a total of 300 to 500 million alveoli within 750 square feet of compressed surface area, the size of one side of a tennis court. To re-create such an efficient apparatus outside the body was almost unimaginable.

During the early 1950s five different medical centers across the country were working on different designs for the heart-lung machine. [4]At Wayne State Medical School in Detroit, Michigan, Dr. Forest Dodrill collaborated with engineers from General Motors. Some thought his machine, the Dodrill-GMR heart pump, resembled a Cadillac V-12 engine. Dodrill's plan was to bypass either the right heart or the left heart for minor heart repairs, thus avoiding the need for an oxygenator altogether. For more complex heart lesions he utilized the patient's own lungs as an oxygenator. Dodrill's original machine, which lacked the versatility of a complete heart-lung apparatus, was used in only four operations before it was abandoned.[5]

The first engineer to work with Gibbon at Harvard estimated that an oxygenator cylinder would have to be about two stories high to provide adequate gas exchange for an adult.[6] Eventually they designed a system of stacked vertical screens that reduced the size of the oxygenator to more manageable proportions. After moving to the Jefferson Medical College in Philadelphia, Gibbon received assistance from IBM engineers. The first Gibbon Model I heart-lung machine was the size of a commercial freezer, weighed over two thousand pounds, and resembled an early-model mainframe computer.

The road to developing a heart-lung substitute to be used during open-heart surgery was littered with flashes of brilliance that often ended in failure.[7] One center used monkey lungs suspended in a glass case to oxygenate the blood, with dismal results. In a method known as cross-circulation, a leading cardiac surgeon used the parent of the child undergoing heart surgery as a human bypass machine. While the overall survival using this technique was better, approaching 50 percent, this procedure doubled the potential mortality from the operation because the parent's life as well as the child's was placed at risk.[8]

From 1951 to 1955, a total of eighteen patients at six heart centers underwent heart-lung bypass-assisted open-heart surgery, and only one survived.[9] Gibbon's first success came on May 16, 1953, with an eighteen-year-old college student who was suffering from heart failure secondary to an atrial septal defect. His plan was to place her on the heart-lung machine so he could patch the hole with a piece of pericardium, but shortly after the pump run began, her blood started to form clots in the oxygenator due to inadequate anticoagulation. With the threat that the machine would cease to function altogether, Gibbon was forced to speed through the operation without a patch. The patient survived the twenty-six-minute pump run, but the case almost ended in disaster.

Three of the first four patients that Gibbon placed on the heart-lung machine died in the operating room, after which he declared a year-long moratorium so that better techniques of diagnosis and management could be developed.[10] Although Gibbon had been the first to successfully close an atrial septal defect with the use of cardiopulmonary bypass, a landmark achievement in itself, he never again performed an open-heart operation. He continued to perform chest operations that did not involve the heart and spent the remainder of his career improving the heart-lung bypass machine.

Encouraged by Gross to try to solve the problem of developing a heart-lung machine to treat newborn respiratory failure, Bartlett collaborated with engineers to design a bypass machine that would allow blood to circulate outside the body (extracorporeally) for longer periods of time. The pivotal component of the invention was the creation of a less traumatic membrane oxygenator that interposed a semipermeable membrane of silicone rubber between the blood and the gas. This solved the problem of the destruction of cells and proteins as the blood circulated through the filter.

Several additional adaptations proved key to the success of the new ECMO technology. The venous reservoir of the heart-lung bypass machine, a large receptacle where the blood was collected, was eliminated, thereby allowing lower doses of heparin to be used. This was a critical advance because neonates were susceptible to intraventricular hemorrhage (bleeding into the brain), especially when fully anticoagulated. Another procedural leap Bartlett discovered was that the blood vessels in the neck—the carotid artery and the jugular vein—were large enough to allow sufficient blood flow during ECMO, so surgeons did not have to use the great vessels of the chest, as required in open-heart surgery. This meant medical personnel could use the bypass machine at the patient's bedside rather than making a trip to the operating room to open the chest.

By 1975, ten years after Bartlett first asked Gross the question, he had built an ECMO machine that would sustain a dog for up to five days at the University of California at Irvine. He had not yet tested the new technology in humans, but one night the neonatologists requested Bartlett's help with a newborn dying from respiratory failure after aspirating meconium-tainted amniotic fluid.[11] The child's mother, an illegal immigrant who was pregnant for the first time, frightened and alone in a foreign country, had driven across the Mexican border in search of a better life for her child. Bartlett met with the baby's mother and explained the procedure along with the difficult-to-quantify risks of a technique that had not yet been successfully used to treat respiratory failure. The mother signed the consent. She then went into the NICU, kissed her daughter, and disappeared, never to be seen or heard from again.

The baby, whom the nurses named Esperanza (Spanish for "Hope"), survived.[12] Bartlett's quest to answer the question of whether a bypass machine could save a baby in respiratory distress was well under way.

ECMO had come into my life when I was a medical student in 1980, when I had barely any working knowledge of the human body and even less practical experience. I was working on a summer research project in the lab of pediatric surgeon Dr. Benjy Brooks. She had just discovered that a heart-lung bypass machine, previously used only for adult open-heart operations, was being developed by Bartlett to treat premature babies with lung disease.

Using bypass to recover the lungs in babies required expensive, specialized equipment and close monitoring of an infant on the pump for several days. The risk of complications, including death, was high, and many doctors were skeptical about adopting this approach. On the other hand, this new therapy, although tested at just one hospital, had shown promise.

Dr. Brooks had seen countless newborns die of lung disease. She knew the sickest were never going to survive without a different approach. This new treatment might be extreme and controversial, but if it had the potential to save lives, she wanted to find out more about it. The best way to do that, she decided, was for our team of three first-year medical students to build a newborn bypass apparatus over the summer and then place a premature lamb on the machine to test it. She hoped that if our animal trial was a success — if the lamb survived — the hospital would fund the effort on a grander scale. She handed us copies of the article and told us to read it and make a list of parts to order.

When she left the room, the three of us looked at each other, bewildered. It was as if she had asked us to build a space shuttle and fly it to the moon. We had sat in a classroom for a year where we were spoon-fed huge volumes of facts on anatomy, physiology, pharmacology, and biochemistry, but we had no practical experience. We had hardly dipped a toe into the vast ocean of medicine, and now we were being asked to construct a sophisticated bypass circuit familiar only to biomedical engineers and heart surgeons.

The article Dr. Brooks had given us to review was written in the foreign language of advanced cardiovascular physiology. What were these *cannulas* and *oxygen extraction ratios*? How would we connect this apparatus to a lamb?

How were we ever going to do this?

Our lack of experience, however, did not deter Dr. Brooks. We were medical students — energetic, inquisitive, bright people. She was sure we could figure this out with some modicum of assistance, so she worked her connections in the medical school and produced a research technician from the cardiovascular surgery department to guide us.

Dave, a bearded, chain-smoking Vietnam vet wearing tinted wire-rimmed glasses, a Hawaiian shirt, and blue jeans, was straight out of a *Doonesbury* cartoon. When he found out what we were trying to do, he rolled his eyes and shook his head. We knew nothing about cardiac physiology and he was way too busy with his own experiments to teach us.

But in the forced marriage that medical school politics regularly engenders, we had no choice, and neither did Dave. We met weekly with him and planned the details of our experiment. He bristled at our basic questions that revealed how little we knew about how the heart functioned in the body. As if tutoring a pack of chimpanzees, he drew diagrams on the board to illustrate simple concepts: how a bypass circuit worked, how it attached to the body, what the complications were.

"In the end," he said, "I will have to put the damn lamb on the machine and it will die and that will be the end of it."

Eventually our parts came in and we assembled the basic circuit—the pump, a reservoir, an oxygenator, and tubing. We assembled a surgical tray with hemostats, forceps, and needle drivers and sent it to sterile processing. We tested the EKG monitor and acquired leads to stick on the lamb. The pregnant ewe arrived, and we prepared for the day of delivery.

When that day came, we waited in pristine scrubs, ready for our big moment. The veterinarian induced the birth early, but a miscalculation had been made. The lamb was more premature than expected, and it stopped breathing within minutes of delivery. With no time to waste, Dave hurriedly inserted tubes into the blood vessels in the lamb's neck and started the machine. But it was too late. We had barely gotten started before the lamb was dead and the experiment was over.

Dr. Brooks walked in outfitted in hat, gown, and mask, fresh from the operating room. We hung our heads as she poked the lamb and took in the scene. This was the moment to dress us down, to confirm our ineptitude in carrying out the project, but those words never came.

She told us instead that this was how it went with medicine, especially when new techniques were at stake. She explained that Dr. Robert Gross, with whom she had trained, had had plenty of failures. Lives were lost as his new surgical techniques were refined. If we were going to be surgeons, we had to have the guts to fail. It was what we turned that failure into that mattered.

What we turned it into pleased Dr. Brooks a great deal. We presented the results of our labor-intensive but unsuccessful efforts at a reception held for the benefactors who had written the checks that supported our research. And when we were finished, they reached into their pockets and purses and wrote more to fund Dr. Brooks's future research projects.

The summer was over and it was time to return to medical school classes. Naively, I thought I was done with ECMO. I had no idea how it would haunt me in the future.

As the hours wore on, it became apparent that Baby X. was heading for ECMO. We had already done the baseline studies — an ultrasound of his brain to rule out hemorrhage, an ultrasound of the heart to look for structural abnormalities, a chromosome analysis to rule out a fatal condition. We had typed and crossed him to determine his blood type and reserved the blood necessary to prime the pump. The next step was to meet with his family, explain the procedure and the possible complications, and get their consent. These discussions were serious because there was only so much that was within our control and the risks were high. It was the early 1990s, when much of the equipment used for ECMO was improvised and the technique was still being refined. There was no getting around the high risk of mishaps and the real possibility that therapy might not be effective.

Still in training, I had already witnessed complications associated with ECMO. I had seen several babies bleed into their brains — a side effect of the blood thinner, heparin. When that happened, the heparin had to be stopped and the baby removed from the pump prematurely, precipitating a rapid decline in oxygen levels and death.

I had seen the kidneys shut down, a not uncommon side effect of a long pump run. When that happened, the body began to swell until the skin became tight, shiny, and blistered. Sometimes we were successful in draining the fluid off with dialysis, and other times nothing we did would reverse the unsightly deterioration that would follow.

I had seen the catheters in the neck pull out, causing blood to spray across the walls and splatter around the baby's bed and onto the floor while someone tried to get a clamp across the spurting ends of the carotid artery and the circuit tubing.

Along with the inherent risks of the procedure, there was the fact that the chances of survival for a newborn with diaphragmatic hernia even with ECMO were still only 50/50 at best. And when a baby had required a patch to close a large defect, like Baby X. had, the mortality was even higher, the worst prognosis of all the conditions we treated with ECMO.

Asking for permission to put a baby on ECMO, especially for diaphragmatic hernia, put parents in a difficult position. On one side of the scale was certain death: *if we continue to ride this ventilator hard, we will enter the home stretch in the rear of the pack, and there is no way we will catch up.*

On the other side, there was a chance of survival, but things could get ugly along the way. Potentially fatal complications might ensue, and the possibility of long-term disability from neurologic injury loomed. Bleeding was a major complication, but using blood thinners was the only way to keep the blood circulating through the pump without clotting the circuit. There was always the threat of intraventricular hemorrhage, or bleeding into the cisterns of the brain where cerebrospinal fluid is produced, especially with premature infants. Other areas of the body might begin to bleed as well—a recent surgical site or the gastrointestinal tract. Another possible complication, because we would have to tie off the carotid artery, was the risk of a stroke that could cause irreversible paralysis and impaired cognitive development.

Parents, listening through a fog of shock and sleep deprivation, could not truly comprehend what they were signing up for. We struggled to prepare them with mere words, knowing that the path ahead was treacherous and could become, in an instant, a horror show. But none of that mattered when their newborn baby was down the hall fighting to live and running out of options.

Despite the risks — death, disability, and a less-than-perfect baby — no parent ever said no to ECMO.

Moments later, Baby X. was prepped and draped. I made a half-inch incision over the midportion of the sternocleidomastoid muscle of his right neck, plunged a hemostat through the belly of the muscle, and split it in two. Two more spreads and the pulsating stripe of the carotid artery came into view. I quickly looped it with a suture and spread deeper. The dark purple bulge of the internal jugular vein surfaced, and I encircled it with another suture.

The pump tech had begun priming the pump and circuit of the bypass machine. He passed off the venous and arterial lines, half-inch-thick tubing that we would connect to the neck cannulas once we got them in. I clamped them to the drapes, turned back to the neck, instructed the nurse to give the heparin bolus, and placed two clamps across the carotid artery. Then I made a three-millimeter incision in the front wall of the artery in between them. My assistant handed me a beveled wire-bound catheter, looking impossibly big for the tiny artery. I wiggled the angled tip through, gently pushed, and slid it all the way down the artery to the arch of the aorta, where it would infuse oxygen-rich blood to the entire body.

Inserting these tubes into a baby's neck was not the most technically demanding procedure in pediatric surgery; nonetheless, it was one that could be dramatic. For example, when you were working on a baby who had just been unloaded from a helicopter with CPR in progress, the brain was oxygen deprived, and every minute counted. The pace quickened from methodical execution to a no-huddle, two-minute drill. We stood by, ready to cut, knowing we had precious few minutes, each of which took a toll in lost brain cells and limited potential.

There were other times when a baby was on a jet ventilator inflating the chest at 360 breaths a minute while we worked on the neck only a couple of inches away, the entire baby pitching back and forth with the constant vibrations. And then there were the technical difficulties, the unpredictable, maddening snags you would hit when you could least afford to, the times when one cannula or the other just wouldn't go into the blood vessel. The plastic tube would taunt you as you twisted, angled, and torqued it, daring you to push harder, but all the while a warning was going off in your head: *if you push too hard, you will tear this tissue-paper-thin vein and ruin it for any future use.*

Getting these cannulas in when a baby was crashing—as opposed to when a baby was stable—was the difference between kicking a field goal in practice when no one was watching and kicking one in the fourth quarter in front of 100,000 hostile fans. The pressure might be rising along with the din of alarms and chattering coworkers, but if you could block out all the auditory stimulus streaming in, the surgical field in front of you would come into sharper focus and the priorities of what must happen next would become clear like the moon on a cloudless night. And then you knew, *This is what must be done to save a life in the next thirty seconds,* and you did it.

Once the arterial cannula was in, I put a rubber vessel loop around the internal jugular to act as a tourniquet, tied off one end, and made a slit in the wall. The venous cannula, even bigger and dotted with numerous side holes along its length, was a little trickier to insert. I twisted it past the first few holes and pushed until it was down inside the right atrium of the heart, where it would drain blood from the body and feed it into the pump to be infused with oxygen.

I took the clamp off the arterial cannula, put my finger over it, watched the blood rise to the top, and clamped again. I carefully inspected the length of the cannula for air bubbles, the tiniest of which could, if they escaped into the body, lodge in the brain and cause a stroke. Air bubbles in a bypass circuit could be deadly, and the entire team inspected the tubing and circuit obsessively for the duration of the ECMO run.

After checking the tubing one last time, I connected the arterial and venous lines to the cannulas exiting Baby X.'s neck. The pump tech started the pump and slowly went up on the flow.

We watched as Baby X. turned bright pink from the top of his head all the way down to his toes.

For the moment, there was still hope.

Through 2010, over 50,000 patients had been placed on ECMO at 150 centers around the world where ECMO was being performed.[13] The majority of patients treated (66 percent) were newborns with respiratory failure, 77 percent of whom survived.

The use of ECMO for newborn respiratory failure peaked during the early 1990s, when approximately fifteen hundred neonates per year were treated.[14] But just as ECMO, an emerging therapy of the 1980s, had burst on the scene in the 1990s by eclipsing older technology, now ECMO itself has had to give way to newer, safer innovations. It has largely been supplanted by interventions that were not as invasive, posed less risk to the patient, required fewer personnel, and were less costly. High-frequency ventilation, for example, which allows rapid, low-pressure inflation of the lungs, was introduced in the early 1990s. Inhaled nitric oxide, a drug that relaxes the pulmonary vasculature, has become a mainstay for the treatment of pulmonary hypertension. Earlier and more regular prenatal care made it possible to begin in utero treatment with steroids to accelerate lung maturity, and shortly after birth, surfactant could be given to premature infants.

But like an organism struggling for survival, mutating from one generation to the next, ECMO evolved into a safer, more efficient, more predictable mode of therapy. The introduction of the dual-lumen veno-venous cannula precluded the need for ligating the carotid artery, thereby decreasing stroke risk. Heparin-coated pump tubing, introduced in the 2000s, supplanted the need for total-body anticoagulation. Amicar, a drug to treat excessive bleeding, became available for patients at risk for a major hemorrhage. Subsequent generations of membrane oxygenators enabled more efficient gas exchange.

Even though the number of newborn ECMO cases has now decreased to about eight hundred cases a year, half what it was at ECMO's peak, the initial success of ECMO allowed an expansion of the therapy into other applications, such as treating older children with respiratory failure from pneumonia, heart patients who need temporary support as a bridge to transplant, and adult patients with respiratory failure. Even now, pediatric and adult ECMO patients have only a 55 percent survival rate, but almost all are patients who would certainly have perished if ECMO had not been available.

Even today with all the safer technologies that have come along for babies, there are still times when nothing can take the place of ECMO.

More than a week later I stood by Baby X.'s bedside, studying the blood pressure and oxygen monitors, scanning the nurse's notes and lab slips, collecting the numbers like I'd done every day for the previous seven days. There was no positive trend, no hopeful sign, nothing to justify the unabated full-court press.

With each passing day that we were unable to wean the baby off the pump even a little, the entire team — nurses, respiratory technicians, and physicians — began to wear looks that all asked the same question. *When are we going to turn it off?*

After such an intense technological tour de force, a huge investment of healthcare resources and hope, we were all discouraged by the dismal outlook. We had stretched the limits of nurses who worked extra shifts as ECMO specialists and were running out of bodies to monitor the pump twenty-four hours a day. The team was worn out, and there wasn't a speck of improvement to spur a second wind.

This was the problem with instituting advanced life support. A bypass machine could keep the patient alive well past the point where it made any sense, past the point where any chance of recovery was likely, and sometimes past the point where normal brain function could be expected. But that point was blurred by how little we knew about the limits of technology and the ability of the human body to withstand physiologic punishment.

Cases like these demonstrated that we knew a lot more about when to turn the machine on than when to turn it off. We could predict when a child in respiratory failure wasn't going to survive without ECMO. We knew when there was no other choice but to go on the machine. And we knew that when a fatal complication developed, like a brain bleed, we would have to shut it down.

What we didn't know was how long to continue a therapy that might never turn things around. Newer technologies, particularly those applied to infants, hadn't been around long enough to have a substantial track record. It could sometimes be hard to know whether we were advancing the ball toward the recovery goal line, but no one ever wanted to give up on a child if there was the faintest hope of recovery.

The mapping of the ECMO frontier was still in progress: what conditions it could treat, which patients should go on the machine. Parameters to assess beginning lung function and predict which patients could benefit from ECMO were still being defined. It would take years to know which patients should have never been put on in the first place, and even now, gray areas persist. In an uncanny sort of way, patients had a way of declaring when it was time to come off by developing complications that mandated it.

Two weeks into the ECMO run, the ECMO specialist pages me just after midnight. She thinks there might be something wrong with Baby X.'s heart. The voltage on the EKG strip is getting smaller and smaller, as if the heart itself is shrinking. She has tried turning up the gain, switching out the monitor, changing the sticky leads on the baby's chest, but the waveform stays the same.

The cardiologist and I arrive at Baby X.'s bedside at about the same time. She is moving an ultrasound probe across the chest over the precordium, the area just to the left of the breastbone where the heart can be palpated. The anatomy has shifted around a bit with the operation, and the ECMO tubes and the heart are not easy to find. Finally she finds it, and the news is not good.

"The heart isn't beating," she says.

"It's not beating at all?" I ask.

"It might be quivering a little, but I wouldn't call that beating," she says.

"Is there fluid around it?" I ask, worried that a fluid collection might be compressing the heart and keeping it from beating properly.

"Maybe a little, but not enough to cause this."

It is two o'clock in the morning, and I need to notify Dr. M., the supervising surgeon. She does not like to hear about problems in the middle of the night, and she especially hates to hear about problems with ECMO patients.

I tell her it looks like the heart has stopped beating, indicating that the patient might well be dead. I wonder if we should take him off the machine. He is not making any progress, and soon we will have to approach the family about ending the treatment.

But Dr. M. is not convinced. She wants me to insert a tube blindly into the space around the heart to see if I can drain out some fluid and get the heart going again.

I wonder at that moment if she is fully awake. Our patient, if not completely dead, is more than halfway there. We have tried everything to revive him. Blood is still circulating in his body, but only because of the pump.

"There must be some fluid in there," she says. "You need to get it out."

I explain to her that the cardiologist sees very little fluid, and how difficult it will be to locate the heart with any accuracy if it isn't beating. There is a high risk I will inadvertently spear it with the sharp end of the trocar inside the tube, which resembles a pitchfork. All I can think is that I will be remembered as the first resident in the history of the training program who has inadvertently impaled the heart. Whether the patient is dead or not, I will be infamous.

"You're not going to hit the heart," she says. "Just be careful."

In the preceding eighteen months, I have never hesitated to do anything that Dr. M. asked, much less refused an order. I am pretty sure, however, that if it is possible to make Baby X.'s situation any worse, this maneuver will do it.

I tell her I can't stick the tube in. I just don't think it's safe, and it would be horrendous to stab Baby X. in the heart on top of everything else he's been through. Either my words finally sink in or Dr. M. thinks I'm the biggest wimp she's ever met, but we decide to operate on Baby X., to open his chest at the bedside and see for ourselves exactly what the heart is doing.

Twenty minutes later we are making a small incision at the level of the xiphoid process, just inferior to the heart. We open a window into the pericardium to drain any fluid that has accumulated, and visualize the heart. By now the EKG is completely flatline, with absolutely no sign of cardiac activity. The pericardium is open. Dr. M. leans in first.

"You're right," she says. "The heart isn't beating." She turns away from the bed, pulls off her gloves, and walks out the door, leaving me to close.

We had called the family earlier, and they were assembled in the very same conference room where, days earlier, in a rush of hope, they gave their permission for ECMO. I explain that the heart is not beating, that we have confirmed this with the exploration. Our options are either to turn the machine off now or allow twenty-four hours more to see if the heart recovers. Either way, the treatment does not appear to be effective. I do not expect Baby X. to survive.

I leave them alone to discuss the options, and walk back to Baby X.'s bed. By now the ECMO specialist has gone home sick, a mix of nausea and disgust no doubt fueling her desire to absent herself. I settle in for what I expect will be another long night, sitting in a chair behind the pump, watching the rollers go around and around, wondering why things like this always happen in the middle of the night and when I will get to sleep again.

And as I'm sitting there watching the rollers of the pump rhythmically spin, barely able to keep my eyes open, the family comes in. They do not speak. They walk up to the bedside, reach up to the canopy, and one by one take down holy cards, rosaries, and photographs of their newborn baby.

They too are ready for this to end.

We hit the power button and it does.

battlegrounds to playgrounds

By the time the four-year-old boy arrived in the emergency room, his heart was still beating, but his body was broken beyond repair. His mother had left him for just a minute to answer the phone in their Harlem high-rise apartment. And that was all it took for him to scramble up to the ledge and tumble, headfirst, out the unscreened window to the sidewalk four stories below.

A short time later Dr. Barbara Barlow was opening the abdomen of her critically injured patient in a Harlem Hospital operating room. His liver was cracked, his spleen was ruptured, but those were the easy parts. She could fix those. What she couldn't fix was his brain. When kids fell out of windows they all landed on their heads, and in this case, the bruising and swelling in his brain would lead inevitably to brain death. She was too late for this little boy, the most recent casualty from the neighborhood. The only way she could have gotten to him in time was if she had kept him from crawling out in the first place.

The thought nagged at her, and it would not go away.

Barlow would continue to witness a constant stream of carnage in her new job as the first full-time pediatric surgeon at Harlem Hospital — gunshot wounds, stabbings, and falls from windows. It was 1975 and she had just finished two years of learning the craft of pediatric surgery in an intensive fellowship that concentrated on congenital anomalies and childhood cancer. Before that she'd spent the better part of a decade operating on sick and injured adults in the Bronx, but this torrent of life-threatening injuries to children was something new to her.[1]

She had never worked in Harlem, though, a place where drugs, violence, and poverty were as pervasive as fog rolling off a harbor in winter. The 1970s have been described as possibly the worst period in the history of Harlem, a time of hitting bottom by nearly ever measure imaginable. Harlem had the highest death rate in New York City courtesy of the glum trifecta of homicide, suicide, and alcoholism. The infant mortality rate, well above average in the late 1960s, doubled in the 1970s.[2] Children openly sold drugs on street corners and joined the ranks of organized crime. There were no jobs and a quarter of families were on welfare. Businesses were shuttered, and three thousand apartments per year were being lost to decay, arson, and abandonment.

No matter your age, your color, or the dreams you held close to your heart, if you were growing up in Harlem your chances of being felled by a major injury were more than twice the national average. Every day trauma ripped families apart, leaving only jagged edges where siblings used to be.

Like it or not, Barlow was in the middle of a war zone. She was willing to operate all day and all night to try and save pediatric trauma victims, but she also began to contemplate what could be done about the relentless gush of wounded blanketing the stretchers in the emergency room.

Barlow realized she needed to step back and consider the bigger picture. A new approach was in order. If she were really going to help the children of Harlem, she should be figuring out a way to prevent injuries from happening in the first place. *Was it even possible? If so, what would it take?* She had no idea, but she knew she had to try.

In the trauma business one learns early about the finality of getting to a patient too late. The first time I saw it, I was an intern on the trauma service. Early one morning, a young woman on her way to work was rear-ended by an eighteen-wheeler. She arrived at the emergency room in shock, her blood pressure dangerously low. A trauma surgeon and I wheeled her straight up to the operating room, as fast as we could move, past hallways crowded with patients on their way to elective tests and procedures, their faces creasing with concern as we barreled through. We skipped the rituals of scrubbing and prepping, pulled on our gowns and gloves, and hustled to the table. The trauma surgeon quickly threw down sterile towels, grabbed a scalpel, and opened her from breastbone to pubis.

Her belly was so full of blood that it flowed out over the edges of the incision, flooded the drapes, and dripped on our shoes below. We had two suctions going just to keep up with it. With so much blood coming out, I wondered how there could be any left in her veins to fill her heart. What would come next? Would the heart cough and sputter like an empty carburetor?

At the head of the table the anesthesiologist worked furiously under the drapes. He started more IVs and hung one bag of blood after another, squeezing them in the palms of his hands until his knuckles blanched.

I learned for the first time the steps you take to get control of massive intra-abdominal bleeding. First we cleared out as much blood as we could, scooping out the clots and sucking up the rest. Then we packed all four quadrants with fistfuls of gauze sponges. This gave the anesthesiologist a chance to catch up, to fill the tank. He pulled out more bags of blood from the cooler on the floor. One after the other he spiked them with the sharp tip of the IV connector and hung them from a metal pole.

We waited, watching the monitors to see when the blood pressure had risen a few points, giving us a cushion between disaster and survival. When it did, we started taking out the packs, one by one, looking for a source of bleeding, something we could patch or tie off.

We pinpointed the problem to the right upper quadrant of the abdomen, behind the liver. Every time we removed that pack, blood welled up like a lake fed by an underground spring. By then it was starting to look like grape Kool-Aid, dark and watered down. Her blood pressure kept dropping, and the anesthesiologist kept giving more blood, but we were losing ground. We finally cleared out enough blood to get to the injury, only to discover that the liver had been pulled out by its roots, leaving gaping holes in some of the biggest blood vessels in the body.

"Forget about giving her any more blood," the trauma surgeon said to the anesthesiologist. "We can't fix this."

Wait a minute, I thought. We can't just give up and let her die. She's still warm. They're still waiting for her at work. How can she be dead before anyone even knows she's here?

Like a linebacker blindsiding a quarterback, the truth knocked the wind out of me. There was a kind of bleeding that surgeons couldn't stop. We were going to have to let her go.

I was not entirely naive. I knew we couldn't cure cancer when it was spreading like measles in a daycare center and had seeded every organ surface in the body. I knew that when a head injury was so bad the white matter oozed out through the ears, there was no way that brain would ever work again. I knew that a flabby, dilated heart, weakened by too many heart attacks, could not be bypassed back to longevity. But up until that moment, I didn't understand you could call yourself a surgeon and watch someone bleed to death.

But patients did bleed to death even within the four walls of an operating room alive with the hum of well-meaning doctors and nurses applying the full-court press of resuscitation and salvage. Patients died because of irreversible shock, because there were limits to what a body could come back from — there were some injuries that simply couldn't be repaired.

I was seeing it for the first time.

Our eyes fixated on the EKG monitor at the head of the bed

watching the heartbeats drift farther and farther apart until there was nothing but a thin green line stretched across a black screen. The surgeon turned away from the table and snapped off his gloves.

"Close her up," he said on his way out the door.

I stood at my side of the table, my hands still resting on the body. It didn't matter whether I used a coarse black silk or a smooth blue monofilament. It didn't matter if my stitches went through all the muscle layers or if I cheated and left out the lining. It didn't matter if she fell apart on the way to the morgue. The only person who would ever see my handiwork was the pathologist performing the autopsy. He would hurriedly snip the thread apart so he could get to the inside, and when he did, he would find the damage we hadn't even tried to repair.

Injury is the leading cause of death from ages one to forty-four and the number one cause of death and disability in children, exceeding all other causes of death combined — more deaths than cancer, heart disease, diabetes, or infection.[3] Motor vehicle accidents account for the majority of childhood deaths, followed by homicide, suicide, and drowning. The order of the specific mechanisms — auto/pedestrian accidents versus car collisions versus auto/bicycle, or all-terrain vehicles — might shift slightly in a given year, but the fact that children die from injury at alarming numbers, approximately 20,000 per year, remains relatively constant, and an additional 50,000 children per year are permanently disabled.[4]

In an era when almost every infectious disease can be treated and vaccinations are given for communicable illnesses, we expect children to be healthy and to survive to adulthood. The fact that injury is responsible for killing the greatest numbers of kids should not, however, be viewed as something we simply must accept. These deaths are not inevitable. And while there is no vaccine to protect against injury, the overwhelming majority of what we call "accidents" are, in fact, preventable events.

But what can be done to prevent an accident? Aren't accidents inherently unpredictable occurrences brought on by misfortune, being in the wrong place at the wrong time? The answer is a surprising no. Populations affected by trauma can be studied to reveal the major public health trends and challenges in a particular state, region, or neighborhood, just as one can uncover the source of infectious disease outbreaks. And just as with any other epidemic, one can put measures in place to slow the rampant spread of casualties.

But first someone has to care enough to do something about them.

When she was a young child, Barlow's father told her, "You're going to be a doctor when you grow up."[5] He himself had taken premed classes before World War I with the hope of becoming a physician, but when he returned injured and too weak to pursue the rigors of medicine, he very openly transferred his dream to his oldest child. After that, the five-year-old Barlow would pull his heavy science texts down from the bookcase and pretend she was in medical school.

In the late 1960s, an era when only 7 percent of physicians were female, Barlow, who excelled academically, initially deferred her dream of entering medical school. Believing she couldn't get in, she detoured into a master's degree in psychology instead.[6]

Later, as a medical student, Barlow became aware that women were generally shunted into one of three acceptable specialties: pediatrics, obstetrics, or internal medicine. After choosing internal medicine, she elected to take a surgical externship in her fourth and final year of medical school to hone her diagnostic skills so she could recognize surgical problems and know when to refer patients.

But something unexpected happened during that pivotal month-long rotation.

"They did me in," she said. "They let me operate."[7]

There were scant female role models in medicine overall, and Barlow had never seen or worked with a woman surgeon. But she had already put her dreams aside once, and, lesson learned, she wasn't going to do it again, forgoing her first choice of specialty simply because of her gender. By the time she realized her change of direction, she was deep into her senior year, too late to apply to surgery programs for the following year.

To correct her errant course, she had to take decisive action. She went straight to the head of surgery at the medical school and explained her predicament. His response was as predictable as the day of the week: *Women should not be surgeons. This is a crazy idea.* She would not even be allowed into the operating room at one particular hospital in the Bronx because the chief of surgery forbade females other than nurses to work there.[8]

But Barlow was prepared for resistance, and instead of taking no for an answer, she offered a compromise. If the chairman would just give her a chance and let her start the program, she would agree to leave if she couldn't meet the demands of surgery residency.

"You just carve me out of the program and I'll go do something else," she told him.[9]

For the next six years Barlow would eat, work, and pick up her laundry at the hospital, totally immersed in surgical training. She had her own room at the hospital and spent every other night there on call — three thirty-six-hour shifts a week. She missed out on movies, plays, books, music, and a social life. She had not expected to have a normal life when she went into surgery, and it never occurred to her to complain.

Her next career decision, however, would introduce an even more substantial hurdle. After years of working in inner-city New York, mostly on adults who were victims of their own reckless habits, the idea of caring for children had begun to take root. Why pediatric surgery?

"Because what happens to children isn't their fault," Barlow later explained. Whether a child was born with a malformation, was hit by a car, or was the unfortunate victim of a serious illness, he was blameless.

If getting into surgery had been difficult, however, getting into pediatric surgery was next to impossible. Of the estimated 375 formally trained pediatric surgeons in the United States and Canada from 1937 through 1973 (the year Barlow would be applying), fewer than ten, a mere 2.6 percent, had been women.[10]

Barlow's interview at the New York–Presbyterian Babies Hospital, where there had never been a female chief resident in any specialty, went as expected: *Was she planning to have children? And what if her spouse became ill? Would she stay home from work and take care of him?*

By the end of it, Barlow was certain she would not be chosen. And she was almost right. She was not the first choice, but when the preferred male candidate changed his mind and walked away from the fellowship, Barlow was still available, and she took the job.

When Barlow finished her training, she was offered a position in private practice, but she wasn't comfortable with the idea of billing patients. She considered becoming a medical missionary instead but then learned that Harlem Hospital, one of the teaching hospitals for Columbia University, where she had trained, was in need of a full-time pediatric surgeon. A cadre of part-time pediatric surgeons were covering the hospital for life-threatening emergencies only, leaving an enormous backlog of five hundred children awaiting elective operations.

Working in the city hospital system, where the majority of patients came from low-income families, appealed to Barlow, and she would never have to bill anyone for her services. She believed kids in Harlem should have access to the same quality of medical care as children from middle-class families. This wasn't exactly the sort of overseas mission she had envisioned when she decided against private practice, but she saw that it would not be necessary to leave the country to apply her skills to the impoverished. In Harlem there was more than enough need.

The pediatricians on staff at the hospital were enthusiastic about her interest in becoming their first full-time pediatric surgeon and wanted to hire her right away, but once again the chief of surgery was saying no to Barbara Barlow. He did not want her hired for the position. He offered her no explanation, but his preference for the current all-male team of part-time pediatric surgeons was obvious. Sexism, a recurring theme of Barlow's early medical career, had reared its head once again, but this time she did not have to talk her way in the door. The pediatricians did the talking for her. They banded together and offered to hire her themselves, outside the auspices of the surgery department.

To the chief of surgery, allowing the pediatricians to hire a surgeon was even worse than hiring a woman himself. He couldn't cede control of his surgeons to another specialty. Recognizing defeat, he surrendered to their wishes and agreed to hire Barlow.

The resistance Barlow met in gaining entrance to the field was not unique. Most women of the era reported similar bias, not only against entry but also in how they were treated even after they were accepted into a residency. Dr. Kathryn Anderson, who later became the first president of the American College of Surgeons (2005), was denied a surgical internship in the late 1960s and pursued a nonsurgical internship instead. When she finally gained admittance to a surgical residency, she was assigned only seven cases during her first two years, compared to a minimum of fifty to one hundred that most junior residents performed.[11]

The 1970s was another lost decade for women in surgery, as only a trickle of women were admitted to surgical residencies. For 140 openings in pediatric surgery across the nation over those ten years, only nine women, including Barlow, were selected. In the larger pool of general surgeons only 5 percent were women. The majority of surgeons were trained in academic medical centers where the chairmen of surgery, all men, were the gatekeepers. There would not be a woman chief of surgery at a major medical school for at least another fifteen years (1987).

Once she was on board at Harlem Hospital, Barlow immediately directed her efforts toward preventing injuries. To do so, she would have to find funding for injury prevention programs, so she started writing grants. She wrote grants for seven years and always got back the same answer: *This is too big a problem for anyone to change. Forget it. Harlem is a resource-limited community, and your group is too small to fix it.*[12]

She found a way to work around the lack of monetary support, recruiting community volunteers to participate in a grassroots effort to decrease injuries. When she started at Harlem Hospital, falls from windows were the twelfth leading cause of childhood deaths in New York City. The New York City Board of Health had recently passed legislation that required landlords to have window gates on all the windows if children age ten or younger lived in the apartment. But the falls continued. Why? Impoverished families, unaware of the law and their rights, weren't notifying landlords that they had young children in the dwelling.

Barlow started working on the "Children Can't Fly" campaign to get the word out. Working through schools and citywide pediatric clinics, parents were given letters addressed to their landlords to include with their rent checks notifying them that a child lived in the dwelling. Once landlords were on notice, they were obligated to install the window guards.

Within a year, the window falls decreased by 96 percent, from an average of twelve patients a year to one. With the campaign's success Barlow had an epiphany. She *could* make a difference in the number of injured coming to the Harlem Hospital emergency room. She saw how effective a simple public health measure, like window guards, could be.

Along the way, Barlow would discover another key part of the injury prevention puzzle, one that would prove to be an invaluable innovation. She teamed up with an epidemiologist at the Columbia School of Public Health to gather hospital discharge and medical examiner data, to set up a population-based injury surveillance system. In this way she would be able to capture injury data on all the children in the community, including those who went straight to the morgue, not just the ones who survived to make it to the Harlem Hospital emergency room.

Armed with statistics, Barlow could document the public health threats to children in the community. She would also need data to prove that a targeted intervention had been successful. She was able to identify injury clusters within New York, and what she found was that the childhood injury rate in Harlem was both twice that of the city as a whole and twice that of the nation. She had suspected this all along, but now she finally had indisputable proof. No one could deny that there was a huge injury problem in the Harlem community.

For years Barlow worked on a shoestring budget, unable to get a major grant, until the Robert Wood Johnson Foundation agreed to provide her with some significant seed money in 1988. With the foundation's support she hired women from the community to help her find out where injuries were occurring and why. She was able to map the community and match street names with specific injuries. She used different colored pushpins—red for gunshot wounds, blue for stab wounds, and yellow for pedestrian injuries—and put them on maps mounted across the walls of her office. Now the injury clusters were clearly displayed for all to see, and the neighborhoods that needed the most attention could be targeted for intervention.

Having data made all the difference in the world. Barlow had suddenly learned the language of change, and that language was numbers. Doors started opening—the mayor, the city council, the commissioners — and everyone started to listen. But now that the problem had been identified, what would she do to fix it? Now that she could truly be an instrument of change, what should she change first?

The answer was staring her in the face. Kids were getting injured because there were no safe places for them to play. Barlow's group had already addressed the danger of falls from windows and made homes safer. But what was happening outside the home? Kids playing in the street were getting hit by cars; kids hanging out on street corners were getting shot. Playground equipment was in disrepair and thus was itself a source of injury. What would it take to create safe places for kids to play?

Further investigation validated Barlow's observation: the one place intended as a safe haven for kids to play, the city playground, was anything but safe. To document that playground equipment violated consumer product safety standards, Barlow's team photographed every park and playground in Harlem. And what those photos revealed was alarming. The parks had been taken over by the drug dealers and the homeless. Broken glass and crack vials were strewn about. The playground equipment was rusty, was missing parts, and had sharp edges that could cut children.

Parents, well aware that parks were not safe, taught children to play in the streets instead. But streets were dangerous places to play too. There was the danger of being hit by a car, caught in gang crossfire, assaulted, or conscripted into a gang.

Barlow's next innovation didn't exactly fit the job description for a pediatric surgeon. Still, she knew it was what she had to do. She would build safe places for children to play.

Modern-day injury prevention is formulated on public health principles — looking at injury the way the spread of a disease might be analyzed rather than attributing it to myths such as "Children are accident prone." When one drills beneath the surface of individual mishaps, it becomes obvious that patterns of injuries are related to specific causative factors within a community, not simply random occurrences.[13]

Much of what we now know about injury prevention is an off-shoot of the initial public heath campaigns aimed at motor vehicle crashes in the 1960s. The postwar economic boom made motor vehicles more available to the public, resulting in an increase in fatalities and injuries from car crashes. Driver error was implicated in over 90 percent of crashes, so initial efforts to decrease fatalities were aimed at training drivers to drive safely. Changing behavior, however, can be difficult.

We take for granted that the vehicles we drive will not crumple or explode on impact, but it was not until Ralph Nader's book about the Chevy Corvair, *Unsafe at Any Speed: The Designed-In Dangers of the American Automobile*, that the debate on car safety was propelled into the public's consciousness. Soon after its publication, the National Traffic and Motor Vehicle Safety Act and the Highway Safety Act of 1966 were passed by Congress and signed by President Lyndon Johnson.[14]

The next pivotal juncture in car safety was the appointment of engineer/physician Dr. William Haddon to head up the National Highway Safety Bureau. When Haddon entered the field, injury prevention was shrouded in the folklore that injuries were the result of "accidents," implying that fate and chance played a role. Haddon insisted on a more scientific approach, like that applied to diseases — one that focused on the causative factors leading up to a particular type of injury. Disease and, by extrapolation, injury prevention could be viewed as occurring in three phases — before, during, and after a human came in contact with a dangerous condition. Just as the causative factors for polio could be identified — the poliovirus, water fountains, and swimming pools — so could the instigators of injury be ferreted out in a community.

Recognizing that human behavior is difficult to control, Haddon moved the injury prevention emphasis from individual behavior to changing the physical environment around the individual. He incorporated the three phases of prevention into an analytical tool referred to as the Haddon Matrix. These criteria help to systematically identify pre-event, event, and postevent interventions involving a human (e.g., the driver), the agent (the car) this human is interacting with, and the environment (e.g., a highway).

The Haddon Matrix, a concept taught in every school of public health, endures today as the premier research tool for how injuries happen and how they might be prevented. It became a model for the prevention of all types of injuries and has recently been used to analyze threats to homeland security such as terrorist bombings and anthrax outbreaks.

Haddon's focus on improving motor vehicles led to the creation of federal standards for automobile design as well as the addition of safety equipment such as seat belts and airbags. His fervent campaigning for improved automobile safety caused him to fall out of favor with some in the automobile industry who found his suggestions excessive and economically burdensome. They forced him out of the National Highway Safety Bureau, but he continued his work at the Insurance Institute for Highway Safety, a nonprofit supported solely by automobile insurance companies. Under Haddon's direction the Insurance Institute became a leader in providing objective information on motor vehicle safety, including crash test ratings on vehicles and researching, evaluating, and educating the public on safety features such as child restraint seats. Courtesy of the work Haddon began, seat belts saved an estimated 255,000 lives between 1975 and 2008.[15]

Haddon blazed the path for those who followed in the field of injury prevention, most notably his colleague Susan Baker, an epidemiologist at Johns Hopkins University. If Haddon was the king of accident prevention, Baker was the queen. In 1968 she was one of the first to ask why so many people (50,000 per year) were dying in car crashes. She wrote to Haddon requesting federal financing for a study to compare drivers who were not responsible for their fatal crashes with drivers who were. Haddon replied with a grant from the National Highway Safety Bureau.[16]

Baker became an indefatigable advocate for protecting the public health and safety through injury prevention, lobbying in person and in her publications for gun control, air bags, motor-cycle helmets, and home sprinkler systems. Recalling her rela-tionship with Haddon, who died an untimely death in his fifties, Baker recited an exchange that took place during a congressional hearing on the passive restraint standard, over which Congress waffled for years.

> After one hearing I asked Bill Haddon, "Do you think we will ever get air bags in cars?" "Sue," he replied, "Go read the his-tory of the battle over milk pasteurization." I did so, and was amazed to learn of the decades of delay. . . . It gave me hope that eventually we would have air bags.[17]

Haddon and Baker drove the injury prevention debate on the macro level, stepping forward as the national mouthpieces for the nascent field, bombarding Congress and the public with irrefut-able data on the dangers of everyday life. Barlow continued her own crusade in the trenches, digging for clues to what was killing the kids of Harlem and preparing to make some waves of her own.

By the late 1980s Barlow's photos of Harlem's playgrounds had gone out to the mayor, the city council, and every principal in the community. And then there was the article on the front page of the *Daily News*—a little girl standing in front of a city park, her hands filled with crack vials. The Commissioner of Parks and Rec-reation showed up in Barlow's office and made it clear. He would do whatever was necessary to improve the parks and to keep any more articles about them out of the paper. He would clean up the city parks, install safe equipment, and create ball fields.

District Attorney Robert Morgenthau joined in the effort and assigned a narcotics task force to the playgrounds. Tipped off by concerned citizens, they went playground to playground, setting up stings to nab drug buyers in the act. New York City had passed a law that allowed the police to seize the car of anyone arrested buying drugs. With the force of the law and the increased attention from the narcotics team, it wasn't long before demand for drugs in the parks dried up.

Barlow did not stop at city parks and playgrounds. Her next target was the schools in Harlem, which had little in the way of outdoor play areas. Most schools had the space for playgrounds, but there was no money to build them. New York City was on the verge of bankruptcy in the 1970s, and what limited resources the school system had went to teachers' salaries and basic supplies. There was no money to fritter away on playgrounds for kids.

The money to install the first school playground should have come from a Department of Health grant written to fund an injury prevention project in Queens modeled on what Barlow had instituted in Harlem. Barlow had pleaded for a small cut of the grant to rejuvenate the playground of the school behind the hospital in exchange for providing strategic advice. She had a vision: at least one entire block in the neighborhood would be a safe block for children. Months later, after the playground had been designed with the help of parents and workers had been hired, the plug was pulled on the funding.

Barlow was incensed. She knew that if the project wasn't funded the community would lose more than just a playground — it would also lose hope. The last thing she wanted was to fail to deliver on a promise. Poor communities were at the end of the line when it came to handouts, and they expected to have promises broken. If the school playground wasn't built, they would never trust her again.

With the help of friends, family, and hospital staff, Barlow raised the money from private donors. At first the money started to trickle in, and then the *New York Times* wrote about the playground project, the first in a city where none of the schools had playgrounds. In response to the article, Barlow started receiving checks and letters from across the country. One generous donor offered to pay for the next playground in its entirety. After that the program took off. The Office of School Facilities for the New York public school system decided it was a good idea for kids to have a place to play after all. There was still no money in the school budget, but they would raise the money through grants if Barlow's group would assist in writing them and in training the schools to plan and implement safe projects the way they had in the first school.

The group assisted in building eight more school playgrounds in Harlem. They teamed up with a playground equipment company to provide the playground components at a discount. Parents and teachers would provide the labor. Kindergarten teachers dug postholes. Mothers and fathers assembled slides and tunnels. Elected officials turned out for photo ops and donated discretionary funds. Eventually school officials met with Barlow's group to review their designs, products, and methods and reached a decision: any further money for school playgrounds in the five boroughs was going through Barlow. In 2008, the amount awarded for school playgrounds was $1.2 million.

At last count Barlow's group had built 110 playgrounds with both public and private money in Harlem and across New York City.

She tackled rusty wrought iron fences that kids were getting impaled on in the neighborhood. She supported and raised money for community members to start two baseball teams, a winter baseball clinic, a soccer league, a hospital-based art program, and the Harlem Hospital Dance Leadership Program.[18] And there would be more playgrounds — one at Ground Zero after 9/11, more in Louisiana and Mississippi after Katrina, and another in Arizona after the mass shooting involving Congressman Gabrielle Giffords, assisted by the Allstate Foundation.

Along the way, it never occurred to Barlow to question whether

her various activities were included in the job description for a pediatric surgeon or any other type of medical doctor.

"Children heal through play," she said.

She had witnessed it in the hospital when kids recovering from major operations trundled off to the playroom bent over and hanging on to IV poles. She had seen it when children joyously scaled the newly installed playground at Ground Zero. Her role had expanded beyond the confines of the conventional practice of medicine, but it had been worth it. By getting kids out of dangerous places and into safe ones she was saving lives.

From 1988 to 1998 major injuries requiring hospitalization decreased by 55 percent for children in Harlem, and violent injuries overall decreased by 45 percent. Another dream of Barlow's had at last been realized. The surveillance system she had helped to put in place shortly after her arrival demonstrated that targeting interventions to a specific type of injury in a particular age group for a given community could decrease injuries. The Harlem Hospital Injury Prevention Program, with two grants from the Robert Wood Johnson Foundation in 1994 and 1998, was able to demonstrate that it could effectively lower injury rates. Barlow's program became the model for the national Injury Free Coalition for Kids, an organization that has successfully replicated her efforts in forty hospitals around the country.[19]

Injury in America, a sentinel report compiled in 1985 by the National Academy of Sciences and the Institute of Medicine, pointed out that injuries were (as they still are) the leading cause of death and disability in the United States among children and adults. Although the number of years of life lost prematurely to injury exceeded the number lost to cancer and heart disease combined, federal funding for injury research was only one-fifteenth that of funding for the latter two.

On the heels of this landmark report, Congress appropriated funds for an injury prevention center at the Centers for Disease

Control (CDC) that put injury prevention on the map. Since then the number of injury research studies has increased dramatically. Have they increased enough? In light of the magnitude of the public health threat that injury poses, some would argue they have not. In the United States nearly 180,000 people die from violence and injuries every year — nearly one person every three minutes. Every year more than 2.8 million people are hospitalized and 29 million people treated in emergency rooms as a result of violence and injuries. Every year violence and injuries cost more than $406 billion in medical care and lost productivity.[20]

Blockbuster Hollywood movies tend to follow a formula referred to as "The Hero's Journey." When first summoned, the hero-to-be refuses the call. But she is inevitably tugged into the action, where she will undergo relentless trials, disappointments, and betrayals. Along the way she will identify her allies and enemies and gain the resolve she needs to face one last hurdle, an obstacle of such magnitude that no mere mortal is expected to surmount it.

The Hero Award, bestowed by the CDC in Atlanta, Georgia, in recognition of major contributions to public health, is not given lightly. Fellow recipients include Rudy Giuliani, the mayor of New York City during 9/11; Dr. Paul Farmer, founder of Partners in Health, a nonprofit network that provides healthcare to the impoverished in developing nations; and former President Jimmy Carter, for leading efforts to eradicate Guinea worm disease. In 2011, pediatric surgeon Dr. Barbara Barlow walked up to the podium at the CDC and received the Hero Award for the work she performed and inspired over the span of her four-decade career to prevent childhood injury.[21]

And like many heroes, Barlow was surprised by the magnitude of her own achievement. "If someone told me that we could prevent child injuries and find the money to rebuild all the playgrounds in central Harlem, I would never have believed them. You never know what you can do until you try."[22]

the weight of the future

"Will the table go any lower?" I asked.

The patient's trunk, large and imposing as a sack of cement, protruded higher than normal above the operating room table. The table height had to be adjusted to accommodate the height of his abdomen; otherwise I wouldn't be able to maneuver the instruments inside it.

"That's as low as it'll go," the anesthesiologist said as he manipulated the controls.

It was still too high. I'd have to stand on a footstool, or maybe two, just to be able to reach inside. After the antiseptic prep I peered down into the cavern of his belly button, one of the deepest I'd ever seen. Sunk inside a four-inch layer of fat was the muscle layer I needed to get to. I grabbed the edges of the pit with two clamps and pulled it up into view.

I cut, looked, but saw nothing but yellow globules of fat. I cut again, still looking for the shimmering white of the fascia that covered the brown fibers of muscle, and there was still no sign of it. I kept cutting and pulling, now excavating through a cavern, my hands slipping from the oily slick leaching out of the thick abdominal wall.

Finally, after about twenty minutes, three times the normal entry time, I was able to push the trocar through and take a look around with a camera. There was more of the same inside, a curtain of fat draped across the intestine, more lining the sidewalls of the abdomen. Like a snorkeler making his way through a dense sea of algae, I moved it around, trying to push it out of my way so I could find the appendix.

"Head down, tilt him toward me," I said.

Now the full weight of the patient's body wedged up against me, dense and heavy, but I needed gravity to help pull the fat out of the way, to clear the path to what I was looking for. After tilting back and forth, up and down, I was able to find it. Tucked inside a layer of fat inside the abdominal wall, the appendix was shrouded in more fat, and inside that fat somewhere there would be blood vessels.

It would take several applications of the laparoscopic stapler, slid through the belly button on a foot-long extension, just to get through all of it. The fatty tissue might slide out of the jaws where the staples gripped the tissue. The stapler might get so greasy it would slide out of the applicator and come apart in pieces. The combination of these technical challenges would add up, one stacked on top of the other, taking more time and increasing the degree of difficulty just enough to throw the operation out of sync.

And the sad thing was, this 175-pound patient was only ten years old.

According to the Centers for Disease Control and Prevention (CDC) childhood obesity has more than tripled in the past thirty years. Approximately 30 percent of children and adolescents are overweight or obese, compared to 60 percent of adults.[1] While there are hopeful signs that the epidemic is starting to level off, it is too early to tell for certain whether it is under control.[2]

The consequences of obesity to a child's health are staggering. The immediate effects include an increased risk of diabetes, high blood pressure, gallbladder disease, fatty liver, bone and joint problems, obstructive sleep apnea, and poor self-esteem. But the chronic payback is even more disturbing. An obese child is more likely to become an obese adult, one who is at further risk for hypertension, coronary artery disease, stroke, type 2 diabetes, osteoarthritis, and an increased risk of breast and gastrointestinal cancers.

Without early, intense intervention, the likelihood of successfully treating childhood obesity diminishes. Children may not be able to appreciate or understand the obesity-related risks in store for them in the future. That is why it is crucial to educate and engage with parents about this critical issue.

For those of us who operate on pediatric patients, the childhood obesity epidemic is particularly noticeable and alarming. This is something that didn't exist when I first entered the field of pediatric surgery in 1990. At that time I rarely operated on a patient who weighed more than my 130 pounds, but over the last ten years, many exceed a normal weight, and at increasingly younger ages.

Not only is the childhood obesity epidemic leading to more operations such as gallbladder removal in children; it's also making the ordinary, everyday operations, like appendectomies and hernia repairs, more difficult. But obesity doesn't just make operations more difficult for the surgeon. It's harder on the patients too. Obese patients are at higher risk from general anesthesia. They tend to suffer more complications after operations. Incisions don't heal as well. Muscles pull apart. Wound infections sprout in the deep layer of subcutaneous fat. Pneumonia and deep vein thrombosis are threats.

Any surgeon will tell you that operating on a thin patient is faster, easier, and safer than operating on an obese one.

After the operation on the young boy, I met with the mother and father in the waiting room. I explained that we had finished the operation and that even though their son's size had presented some challenges, I expected him to recover. He might still develop a wound infection or some other complications, but we would be watching him closely.

Then I asked the question. Had they noticed that their son was overweight?

"We are big people, Doctor," the dad said, "but we are worried about him."

He went on to explain how they had started walking after school for exercise and trying to make healthier meals at home, but it was hard to control what their son ate, especially when he was at school or visiting friends or relatives.

I had learned that in talking with families about obesity, treading lightly, simply introducing the topic, was usually enough to get the parents to open up. They voiced their struggles, frustrations, and mounting concerns as the weight kept increasing. Striking the right balance between being overly critical or too permissive was not easy for parents and left them grasping at solutions, hoping to find some way to make a difference.

What could they do? If I would only tell them what to do, they would follow my instructions. How could they help their son get the weight off?

And now we were facing the heart of the problem. There was no obvious solution, no magic bullet or surefire recipe to losing weight when a child had been gaining over a period of years and had easy access to junk food. Food had become a comfort, a habit. For this child to now lose weight, his health would need to take center stage in the family. Everyone was going to have to learn to eat differently. Everyone would have to make a commitment.

There weren't many success stories to draw hope from, but one stood out in my mind—the story of twelve-year-old Marshall Reid reported in the *New York Times*.[3] Marshall, bullied about his weight for years, made the decision to do something about it the day a classmate bluntly told him, "You're fat." He went home that day and constructed a thirty-day plan, a takeoff of the movie *Supersize Me*, but instead of eating at McDonald's every day, his family would eat healthy food.

"We can call it 'portion size me,'" Marshall proposed. Before long Marshall was featured cooking healthy meals in YouTube videos, and eventually he coauthored a book with his mother, *Por-*

tion Size Me: A Kid-Driven Plan to a Healthy Family, which detailed his plan including recipes. Along the way his body mass index (BMI)[4] decreased from 32.3 to 27.4 and he dropped two pant sizes.

Written from a kid's point of view, Marshall's book delivered an inspiring message that everyone could understand: *I might be just a kid, but I've taken responsibility for my weight and the changes I need to make.*

I kept copies of Marshall's book in my office and gave the family a copy the next day.

Parents always want to blame themselves for their kids' problems, as Marshall's mom initially did. She made excuses for his weight, expecting him to grow out of it just as his father had at that age. She didn't cook enough. She let Marshall eat bags of caramel corn in the car. With his father deployed overseas, she was too permissive.[5]

But Marshall's older, soccer-obsessed sister wasn't overweight. So who or what was really to blame? As it turns out, there is no simple answer to this question: kids are exposed to numerous messages about food, not just from parents and siblings but also at school, from friends, and, most particularly, from television.

At the Yale Rudd Center for Policy and Obesity, Dr. Kelly Brownell has honed in on what he believes to be the primary cause — the food industry. "When the history of the world's attempt to address obesity is written, the greatest failure may be collaboration with and appeasement of the food industry," Brownell has written.[6]

Brownell has spent decades trying to bring his message into the government's and the public's consciousness. He has coauthored studies that exposed the poor nutritional content of foods aimed at the pediatric market, especially cereals. He has served on panels, written books, and published papers. He continues to worry, however, that too little is being done to address the childhood obesity epidemic. He believes we will look back at this period of history and wonder why more wasn't done, why we were taking baby steps while our nations' children were being ravaged by obesity, why we didn't do more to stop this epidemic like we would any other.

In the midst of all the other health initiatives that have gained momentum in the United States over the last twenty years — the antitobacco surge, Mothers Against Drunk Driving, improved highway safety — one wonders how the obesity epidemic stayed under the radar for so long. By most estimates it's been taking root for the past thirty years. It's almost as if we walked out into the street one day and there were suddenly twice as many obese people walking around as the day before.

Investigative reporter Michael Moss recently shed light on how the origins of the obesity epidemic were rooted in a food industry that systematically assaulted the American public, particularly kids. The increased intake of sugar-, fat-, and salt-infused foods had been carefully planned and implemented by the "game-changers" — food engineers who knew how to tinker with appetite and satiety. Consumers were induced to eat excessive amounts of food that would never quite fill them up, thereby driving them to eat more. Instead of a nourishing, life-sustaining substance, food was becoming toxic. Recognizing that obesity was becoming a major public health issue, food industry scientists first began to sound the alarm in 1999. The obesity epidemic could place political pressure on the food industry to change its marketing strategy toward kids.[7]

Now everyone is in a panic about childhood obesity. At least ten new articles a day pop up in Google searches, originating everywhere from New York City to the smallest towns in America. By 2012, everyone from doctors to celebrities and famous athletes, from First Lady Michelle Obama to academics — in short, everyone with a platform — was sounding the alarm about this newly discovered epidemic.

But when we take a minute to step back and contemplate the

world we inhabit in 2014, no one should be all that surprised that this has occurred. Society as a whole has written the perfect script for obesity to run wild, disseminate like the plague, and prey on our children.

There is a simple formula for weight gain: the amount of calories consumed exceeds those expended in the course of a day. From 1980 to 2010, the American public was bombarded with cheap, high-calorie food, and by 2012 the average American adult was consuming three hundred more calories a day compared with thirty years ago.[8]

Fast food, dense with fat and carbohydrates, exploded into our daily lives. McDonald's stock was booming worldwide, with outlets metastasizing even to hospitals. Junk food wasn't just sold in restaurants and grocery stores. It was sold everywhere — gas stations, schools, and drug stores. A soft drink vending machine morphed into the dispenser of an array of drinks, snacks, and quick-serve meals. But it didn't stop there — food became an appendage to every business a person walked into. New social customs developed around food: breakfast tacos for coworkers, after-school practices with parent-supplied snacks, corporate meetings with cookies and lattes. Food, lots of it, was always available.

Sugar-laden soft drinks ballooned from large to extra large to the giant forty-five-ounce "Big Gulps." Cereals, candy, and fast food were marketed to kids on television, online, and even through cell phones. Restaurants served value meals with oversized portions, and all-you-can-eat buffets dotted the landscape of American cities.

The fact that people eat more when they are served more is known as the Portion Size Effect. Studies have shown that people will eat up to 25–50 percent more than usual if served more. We also tend to consume food in units. Our perception is that whatever comes in a bag, bottle, or box is the appropriate size for a single serving.[9]

On the activity side of the equation, Western society has been completing our conversion from active humans who worked the land, walked, and played outdoors to an almost completely sedentary society. By the year 1990, people were spending, on average, ten hours a day or more sitting, whether in cars commuting from greater and greater distances, in classrooms, or at the job or in front of a screen of some type. Many children no longer had the option of school-based physical education, as these classes were the first to be cut when budgets got tight. In two-parent households both parents were heading off to work every day, leaving scant time for meal preparation. Microwave-ready processed foods and restaurant takeout became embedded into family life. People ate out more. Kids were left on their own to order in pizza.

Sustained movement was no longer necessary in daily life. The only way people would get exercise was by consciously planning for it. We became — and remain — a nation of overconsuming mammals who barely move, which is why the obesity epidemic shouldn't have been a surprise. This epidemic was inevitable.

It is difficult to contemplate the future healthcare costs of obesity without launching into a full-scale panic. Being obese raises a person's healthcare spending by 36 percent, a higher rate of increase than smoking or alcoholism — approximately $2,700 to $3,000 more a year for an obese individual than a nonobese person.[10] Obesity-related medical costs total $190 billion a year, equal to 20 percent of all healthcare spending, over half of which comes out of the federal healthcare budget in the form of Medicare and Medicaid spending.[11]

But the economic costs of obesity are not just from treating the medical complications. Lost worker productivity and absenteeism from the job are also costly to employers. As a person's BMI increases, so do the number of sick days, medical claims, and healthcare costs. This alone has prompted employers to promote weight management programs at work and, in some scenarios, to limit or ban the hiring of significantly overweight employees.

The fact that the overweight and obese are frequently the targets of discrimination has raised the question of how pervasive weight bias is in our society. Studies have shown that overweight individuals face discrimination when seeking employment. Performance evaluations and salary are affected by weight. This bias pervades the educational system, where overweight and obese students face weight discrimination from teachers, peers, and parents. Expectations for academic achievement are lower, and anti-fat attitudes are informally endorsed.

In a study of family practitioners, their own treating physicians viewed overweight and obese patients as awkward, unattractive, and less compliant. Medical students and nurses share these negative views. The majority of physicians feel ill equipped to counsel patients regarding successful weight loss strategies and believe that weight loss efforts are bound to fail.[12]

Weight bias can, in fact, be found across most segments of society. Overweight and obese characters are stigmatized in television and film and stereotyped in cartoons and videos aimed at children, which often depict such characters as unattractive, slovenly, or less educated, a phenomenon known as "fattertainment."[13] In the Harry Potter series, for example, Potter's obese cousin Dudley is portrayed as dim-witted, greedy, and mean, as are Dudley's parents.

Television shows like *The Biggest Loser*, *More to Love*, and *Celebrity Fit Club*, which exploit an entire cast of obese individuals who are desperately trying to become thin, can't help but subject them to shaming and ridicule when weight loss goals are not met. It is no wonder, then, that the overweight and obese are susceptible to depression, low self-esteem, and poor body image, consequences that fuel the risk for further weight gain and the avoidance of physical activity.[14]

This phenomenon of weight bias has spurred the Rudd Center at Yale to create an image gallery with a collection of photos that portray obese individuals in a positive way. The Obesity Action

Coalition is a nonprofit that represents the obese advocating for accessible education and treatment as well as promoting entertainment options that show obese individuals in nonstereotypical settings, such as successful doctors, lawyers, and action heroes.[15]

When I walk through an airport, I can't help noticing the juxtaposition of overweight Americans with endless offerings of processed, unhealthy food. Once I am through security and en route to my gate, I will pass barbecue, cinnamon rolls, pizza, tacos, ice cream, cookies, more ice cream, and the ubiquitous McDonald's.

Airports have become food emporiums.

I will duck into the bookstore seeking respite in newspapers and paperbacks only to find more food — candy bars, oversized sodas, nuts, chips, cookies. They are even selling junk food on the plane.

But in this same place, surrounded by all the trappings of the obesity epidemic — the numerous vectors and victims — there is no mention of the elephant in the room: a physically disadvantaged population destined for chronic diseases making itself sicker by overindulging. If someone was overdrinking in an airport bar, there would be a point at which a bartender would no longer serve him or her, but with food no such limit exists. If people want to gorge themselves with two hot dogs, a cinnamon roll, and a bowl of ice cream, they can do so unfettered by society or the law.

We force passengers to line up in various states of undress to screen for guns, knives, and explosives because of the remote, theoretical risk of a terrorist attack. But we do not screen high-risk individuals for obesity, a much more imminent threat. We do not even hand out educational material about the dangers of obesity or healthier food choices. Instead we abet the epidemic with more junk food per square foot than one could ever find on any city street. In the midst of one of the largest public health crises in decades, we do nothing.

Mary, a fifteen-year-old girl referred for gallbladder removal, has been having pain under her ribcage on the right side, off and on, for about six months. The pain is worse after meals. She doesn't have gallstones, the more traditional, indisputable indication for gallbladder removal, but her gallbladder is not functioning normally. A HIDA scan, a study that measures how the gallbladder is emptying, shows that her gallbladder is contracting at less than 20 percent of capacity. It is likely crammed with cholesterol from a diet high in fat and low in fiber. The gallbladder should be excreting bile, but the bile can't squeeze past the thick pastelike sludge blocking the outlet to the gastrointestinal tract, and when the gallbladder contracts it causes pain. Mary is not obese, but she is overweight, and her diet is packed with junk food and fat.

I bring up the notion that even though she has been referred for gallbladder removal, there are other alternatives. We could put her on a diet, one low in fat and high in fiber, to try to avoid an operation and save the gallbladder.

Her mother looks at me askew.

"Why save it?" she wants to know. "Why save something that is nothing but a source of pain? In our family gallbladders are removed early—grandmother, aunts, cousins."

It's as if they expect to lose this bothersome organ, the gallbladder, as sure as they do baby teeth, as if it has no useful function at all.

But it doesn't have to be that way.

There are good reasons to keep the gallbladder. While a person can live without one, and thousands do, the gallbladder has a function in the body. As the liver produces bile, a detergent-like substance that aids in digestion, the gallbladder stores it. After eating, bile is released into the first portion of the intestine. Without a gallbladder, bile drips nonstop into the intestine 24/7.

This is not how digestion was designed to work. Some patients suffer side effects after gallbladder removal, like severe diarrhea, excessive gas, or indigestion. Studies have suggested that the constant drip of bile may injure the intestine or predispose it to malignancy.

Since Mary does not have gallstones or definite indications for removal, I recommend a trial of dietary therapy to see if her symptoms will go away without surgery. But her mother is resistant to this course of action. She tells me again: *these bad gallbladders run in the family, and it's Mary's turn.*

Mary is silent.

Her mother will be disappointed if I don't take Mary's gallbladder out. She brought Mary in today to get the operation scheduled, and in her mind this will be a wasted visit if she leaves without a surgery date in hand. But this is also an opportunity for Mary to start living a healthy lifestyle, to make a change in her eating habits that will affect the way she lives the rest of her life. If I take Mary's gallbladder out and her pain goes away, she'll feel better for a while. But if the pain recurs or if Mary keeps eating high-calorie junk food and eventually becomes obese, have I done her any favor? I realize in standing my ground that Mary and her mom might leave my office, walk down the street, and find another surgeon who will be only too happy to yank this gallbladder out and toss it into a shiny pan, but that's their choice. I tell them we should try some other solutions before operating.

I've taken an informal survey of my colleagues to find out who believes that decreased gallbladder contractility is real pathology. *Who takes out a normal gallbladder when there are no stones? I'm just curious. Is everyone drinking the Kool-Aid?*

Never on the first visit, one says. *I put them on stool softeners, treat them for constipation, and see them back to see how they're doing.*

If they're obese, I make them lose weight first, another colleague advises. *If they start losing the weight, the pain usually goes away.*

Never. I never take out the gallbladder if there are no stones, a different surgeon weighs in. *I just don't believe poor gallbladder function is the real issue, and I don't want to perform unnecessary operations.*

All across America, surgeons are removing the gallbladders of overweight and obese children because of an abnormal HIDA test, a somewhat recent and, some believe, equivocal indication. The gallbladders of patients with poor emptying due to a high-fat diet may look perfectly normal at operation. Why are we taking out something that looks normal?

I review the medical literature to find out if the data supports taking out all these gallbladders. Gallbladder removal in childhood in this country has been increasing at an alarming rate over the last decade, and the majority of that increase is in overweight or obese children. Thirty percent or more of children who have their gallbladders out will continue to have abdominal pain. Seventy-five percent of patients with abnormal HIDA scans have marked improvement in abdominal pain two years later whether they had their gallbladders removed or not.[16]

There is perhaps no better example of the failure of our healthcare system as a whole than the unchecked rise of the childhood obesity epidemic and this gallbladder removal phenomenon that has come along with it. American physicians are trained to treat disease and are rewarded financially for doing so. Preventative medicine, where the focus is on keeping the patient healthy, takes a back seat to testing, diagnosing, and treating illnesses. Newer generations of physicians will likely be better educated in preventative medicine principles, and hopefully they will pay more attention to addressing excessive weight gain at all ages.

The childhood obesity epidemic didn't happen overnight. It was germinating for at least two decades, years when patients were still seeing their doctors for annual visits, supposedly being weighed year in and year out, and every year they got bigger.

What can ultimately be done about an epidemic that is brought about by the pervasive creep of a harmful lifestyle that people choose for themselves? The cause of the childhood obesity nightmare is still being unraveled, but what has become apparent is that government intervention is essential to putting the brakes on the runaway train.

Will Americans eat healthier if they have the choice? Amazingly enough, the fast food industry pitched leaner, healthier choices to the American market in the early 1990s, only to be disappointed in the results. In 1991, McDonald's rolled out the McLean Deluxe hamburger, a beef/seaweed extract hybrid with only 9 percent fat, less than half of their typical patty, but it was a huge flop.[17] The same fate followed for Wendy's, which trialed a lighter menu in 1985, including a tomato half stuffed with tuna, cottage cheese, and pineapple salad on lettuce.

The public wasn't interested.

"We spent a whole year and about $10 million advertising this menu and nobody would bite," said Wendy's spokesperson Dennis Lynch.[18]

A light pizza marketed by Pizza Inn failed too. Chicken sandwiches were the one menu item marketed as health food that did make the cut and today remain a popular choice.

In recent years, federal, state, and municipal governments are relying less on consumers to make the healthy choices and instead are moving forward with eliminating the more unhealthy ones. That is, they are trying to legislate common sense, and this is not always being greeted with enthusiastic support by the masses.

New York City tried to ban sugar-sweetened beverages (SSBs) larger than sixteen ounces from restaurants, movie theaters, and street carts, before the law was overturned in court.[19] SSBs have been viewed as one of the major bad actors of the fast food binge, not only because they deliver enormous quantities of sugar and no nutritional value but also because SSBs are not nearly as effective in suppressing appetite as solid food. Policy makers have proposed a national tax of a penny per ounce on SSBs to offset the healthcare costs of obesity and to discourage their consumption.

Citing links between trans fats (partially hydrogenated oils) and coronary artery disease, the Food and Drug Administration (FDA) has recently taken steps to ban trans fats from food.[20]

New federal regulations now require operators of restaurants with twenty or more stores to post calorie counts in the hope that consumers will choose healthier options. No one knows for certain how big an impact this will have on consumer behavior. Early studies have been mixed, with some showing a shift to lower calorie choices and others detecting no change in behavior at all. One recent study found that restaurants that had increased lower-calorie menu items experienced an average 5.5 percent increase in sales, compared with a 5.5 percent decrease among chains offering fewer lower-calorie servings.[21]

In 2012, the Robert Wood Johnson Foundation published a study measuring the trend in obesity rates from 2007 to 2011 that finally showed a ray of hope in the ongoing three-decade epidemic. New York City reported a 5.5 percent decline, Philadelphia reported a drop of 4.7 percent, and Los Angeles saw a 3 percent decline. Mississippi, with one of the nation's highest childhood obesity rates (41 percent), reported a 13.3 percent drop.

A common theme among successful cities was the implementation of comprehensive programs that targeted schools and communities in promoting healthier eating and increased physical activity. New York City was particularly aggressive: it was among the first to ban trans fats from restaurants; to require daycares to offer exercise, adhere to nutrition standards, and limit television time; to require fast food restaurants to list calories, and of course to ban huge sodas.[22]

While there are encouraging signs that at least the increase in obesity has leveled off, we cannot afford to become complacent about childhood obesity. As a society, we — parents, physicians, and schoolteachers — fell asleep at the switch as the childhood obesity epidemic rolled along. We all have to step up, because as this generation matures into adulthood they are projected to develop coronary artery disease and type 2 diabetes in staggering numbers and at the youngest ages ever recorded. Any hope of reining in healthcare spending will be lost if this disaster scenario unfolds.

Knowing the devastating lifelong effects of obesity and the high (up to 60 percent) failure rate of behavioral treatment, the question arises, how aggressive should we be at treating the children swept up in this epidemic? Approximately 220,000 adults undergo weight loss surgery a year, yet currently only 1 percent of all weight loss operations are performed in children.[23] Does this make any sense in light of the urgency of the problem and the future impact on a child's health?

There are overriding factors to consider when contemplating a weight loss operation on a child. Weight loss operations are, by definition, elective rather than urgent operations. They alter a child's anatomy and digestive function, some more than others. They may have lifelong implications and side effects, such as the inability to tolerate full meals, diarrhea, or digestive problems.

Some take the stand that if we don't allow children to sign up for elective plastic surgery, why would we allow them to undergo a weight loss operation that might have lasting consequences? We should at least wait until a child had decisional capacity (estimated to be age thirteen) and can truly understand what he is signing up for over the long term. Some obese children, in the range of 30 to 60 percent, will somehow manage to overcome their weight issue by the time they reach adulthood.[24] If every child who met the criteria for operation had one, at least some portion would have been unnecessary over the long term.

Another consideration is that children are still growing and require certain nutrients to do so. A weight loss operation might curtail the supply of nutrients essential to proper growth and development. Complicating matters even further is that insurance companies have a history of not covering the costs of weight loss surgery in children as they do in adults. Medicaid in almost every state will now cover bariatric surgery in qualifying adolescents, but the same is not necessarily true of insurance companies. Citing safety and efficacy concerns, many plans have the policy of covering only patients eighteen and over. As more information is gathered about the costs of treating childhood obesity victims over the course of a lifespan, these barriers are likely to fall because despite the inherent concerns raised by performing them in children, weight loss operations are the only thing left to try when lifestyle control fails, as it frequently does. For those most severely affected the future is otherwise dim.[25]

Because of these concerns, stricter criteria are recommended when considering bariatric surgery on adolescents.[26] First, children must be severely obese, with a BMI greater than 40 or have serious obesity (BMI > 35) and at least one major obesity-related disease such as diabetes or heart or liver disease. Patients must be close to their expected adult height. They must have failed at least six months of organized weight management programs, have decisional capacity, be willing to undergo psychological evaluation, and, in the case of females, agree to avoid pregnancy for at least one year after the operation. They must also be willing to adhere to nutritional guidelines postoperatively — that is, agree to eat smaller, healthier meals — in order for the operation to be successful.

Despite seemingly overwhelming odds against obese kids, occasionally I do see signs of hope on a case-by-case basis. Two weeks after that 175-pound patient had his appendectomy, he and his mom came in for a postop visit and excitedly shared the news: they're counting calories at home and already seeing the results.

Will it last? I don't know. They could get distracted, lose their enthusiasm, and get discouraged if the weight loss levels off. But this family is at least pointed in the right direction, with the hope that this one child will be able to change a future that had veered toward medical complications and a shortened lifespan. He can't afford not to change, and we can't afford not to help him.

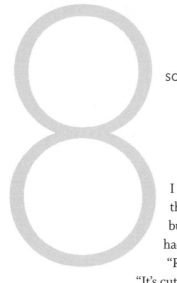

something to celebrate

I couldn't help but notice. I hadn't seen them in several months, maybe six or so, but the last time I saw Rachel's mother, she had had a full head of hair.

"Rachel shaved it," she told me.

"It's cute," I said.

I glanced at her daughter's own hairless head. Only a few wisps of solitary hairs remained at her neckline and around her ears. Her mother's appearance needed no further explanation. I knew it was one of those things that mothers do for daughters, especially five-year-old daughters who have lost all their hair to chemotherapy.

"I was a movie star for Halloween," Rachel blurted out.

Her mother proudly whipped out a hefty stack of glossy photos. Rachel was posing boldly for the camera, her hands held high above a full head of teased red hair. She sported a shimmering evening gown, comically risqué for a child. A wide ribbon of lipstick blotted her mouth, and she had eyebrows again, drawn in by her mother, for the first time since her treatment began.

Rachel was being treated for rhabdomyosarcoma, a highly malignant tumor that originated in the muscle tissue of her back. In the continuum of cancer that extends from favorable to unfavorable to just plain horrible, Rachel's type would fall into the not-so-great end of the spectrum. At the first operation the tumor had been large and fixed, spreading diffusely throughout the tissues, so only a biopsy was performed. Sometimes tumors, particularly large ones, may be too close to vital organs or other structures that, if removed, would cause long-term disability. In such cases a surgeon may opt to biopsy the tumor, have the pathologist identify exactly what type of tumor it is, and then determine the optimum treatment plan.

To shrink the margins of the tumor and control the spread of it throughout her body would require several rounds of some of the strongest chemotherapy available, her only hope for cure. So Rachel underwent another operation just to put in a Broviac catheter, a long white tube that was tunneled beneath the skin of her chest, under her clavicle, and guided into a large vein, where it ultimately rested just inside the heart. This catheter would minimize the number of sticks Rachel had to endure for countless blood draws and ensure that caustic chemotherapy drugs were delivered directly into the bloodstream.

Most of us think of cancer as a disease of adults, a devastating diagnosis our friends, neighbors, and coworkers get hit with in the prime of life. We are jarred when someone we know in their thirties, forties, or even fifties receives the news of what could be a terminal diagnosis. The idea of a child having cancer is even more unsettling, but approximately 12,000 children in the United States are diagnosed with it each year.[1] The peak incidence of childhood cancers is in patients under two years of age. When compared with adults, childhood cancer only comprises 2 percent of all cancer cases; however, it accounts for 10 percent of all deaths among children and is the leading cause of death from disease in children.[2]

While we never fail to be shocked and saddened when a child is diagnosed with cancer, there is some comfort in the fact that we expect many, up to 80 percent, to be cured, compared to only 65 percent of adults.

Why do kids with cancer fare better than adults?

The number one factor is the fact that pediatric cancers are biologically different from adult cancers. While childhood cancer shares some similar characteristics to adult cancer — it can spread, come back months to years later, and be fatal — in many respects it is almost a different disease. The most common adult cancers — skin, prostate, lung, breast, and colon — are frequently linked to long-term exposure to carcinogens such as the sun or tobacco and are seldom seen in children. Adult cancers are derived from cells that line cavities and glands, known as epithelial-type cancers.

Childhood cancers are derived from embryonal, or immature, tissue types originating from nerves, brain, bone marrow, bone, and muscle. As is true for any cell type undergoing relatively rapid cell growth, childhood cancer types are in general more responsive to chemotherapy and radiation than adult types of cancer are. The most common cancers in childhood, making up 50 percent of all childhood tumors, are leukemia and brain tumors. Neuroblastoma (a tumor of nerve origin found in the chest or abdomen), Wilm's tumor (a type of kidney cancer unique to toddlers), and lymphoma make up the bulk of the rest. In addition to possible toxic exposures such as in utero radiation, childhood tumors may be linked to errors of normal embryologic processes or genetic disorders.

The second major factor affecting outcome from cancer treatment is that children are more resilient to the side effects of cancer treatment. Children are less likely to have chronic diseases such as diabetes, heart disease, or liver or kidney impairment, all of which can affect how a person metabolizes chemotherapy and how toxic the drugs are to the body. Certain chemotherapeutic agents are more toxic to individual organs and limit how much of a specific drug can be administered.

The third factor is that a specialized network of pediatric oncologists, who pool their results in a cooperative and collaborative manner, administers the majority of childhood cancer treatment. Pooling the data allows researchers to follow trends more closely, to determine what treatments are most effective for children, and to adjust drug doses with the goals of limiting toxicity while still achieving cure. This system developed over time because pediatric cancers occur in such small numbers compared to adults, making it more advantageous, and in fact necessary, to pool data in order to establish any meaningful trends. More than 60 percent of children are enrolled in clinical trials, versus only 3 percent of adults.

Kids with cancer have one other huge advantage over adults that is of paramount importance. Their primary caretakers are almost always their parents. Parents have a unique stake in the health of a child, someone they value above all else. They seek out the best treatment possible for their children, even more so than for themselves. Parents make sure children make it to their doctor's appointments and take their medications, that they continue to eat and drink even when they don't feel like it. Parents are there every day and around the clock when necessary. They call the doctor when something doesn't look right — for example, when their child might be experiencing a side effect of treatment such as fever or vomiting — and bring them back to the hospital quickly if their condition worsens. Very few adults have such dedicated caregivers as the built-in ones kids do. Does it make a difference? Those of us who treat kids believe that it does.

There is nothing easy about cancer treatment. It involves cutting, scanning, poisoning, and radiating the body for months. The success of the therapy is frequently not known until months or years afterward. Along the way, patients are so nauseated they can't eat for days. Their hair falls out. They become fatigued and lack the energy for extended play. There's a good chance they'll suffer at least one life-threatening complication that will require a prolonged hospitalization, and if they live long enough after it, the treatment itself can cause secondary cancers to develop in the body, can retard growth, or can even result in permanent disability like the loss of a limb, an eye, the use of a hand.

The intensity of cancer treatment is a difficult construct for most people to grasp until they go through it. Try selling it to a child who may not fully understand what this thing "cancer" is and why, all of a sudden, it has shown up and changed everything.

When faced with the prospect of a serious illness, kids don't ask the same questions that adults do. They don't ask about chances for cure or side effects. They want to know how much the next procedure's going to hurt and whether they'll be awake for it. They ask how big the scar will be, when can they get in the pool, whether they'll have to miss next Saturday's soccer game.

Kids live for today.

But for parents who are threatened with the loss of a child, everything changes in an instant with the diagnosis of cancer. They move from shock to tolerance and eventual acceptance of what their child must endure to have even a chance at survival. They cancel vacations, rearrange work schedules, take out their calendar and begin to schedule and negotiate endless clinic appointments and unexpected hospitalizations. Soon the gravity of the illness weighs on every member of the family. Life has been put on hold.

And then there is the rare person like Rachel's mom. There is no way around the pain of being poked, the unsightly scars and the missed birthday parties, but if there was any fun to be had in all this, she was going to find it. Rachel was distracted with a constant stream of activities — clown shows, cooking lessons, craft projects, and parties — enough to make up for all those that were missed and more. Even on the inevitable bad days when Rachel had to go into the hospital for infections and get stuck for ivs and blood tests, there was always something fun to anticipate when the dark cloud lifted. Rachel's mother kept planning and doing and wishing for the best, and so, by example, did Rachel.

Today there are three basic ways to treat cancer — surgical excision, radiation, and chemotherapy. Cancer treatment in the

1940s, however, was a two-dimensional system dominated by radical surgery and supported by a primitive version of modern-day radiation therapy.

With very little else in the toolbox the best chance for curing any cancer was to get it out early, before it had spread outside the organ of origin. It was not enough simply to remove a tumor. A rim of normal tissue known as a "clear margin," forming a boundary between the abnormal cancer cells and the normal body tissue left behind, was included in the resection. Having a clear margin was an essential step in preventing tumor recurrence. Immediately after a tumor was removed in the operating room, the correct anatomical orientation was marked with sutures to indicate the north, south, east, and west borders of the tissue mass, and it was sent to the surgical pathology lab while the surgeon, still scrubbed, waited for the report.

The pathologist would stain the boundaries with India ink and perform frozen sections on the tumor margins to verify that there was a margin of normal tissue and that there were no active tumor cells left behind in the patient. If a particular margin was positive, the pathologist would relay the information back to the operating room and the surgeon would cut out more tissue, if possible, and send it back to the pathologist to once again inspect the margins.

Excising the tumor en masse did not mean that microscopic cancer cells had not already leached into the lymph system or bloodstream and colonized a distant site in the body. For this reason even more radical surgeries were designed to dissect out and remove lymph nodes with the specimen.

The radical mastectomy for breast cancer was one such example of a radical cancer operation: the entire breast and overlying skin were excised, along with the lymph nodes under the arm and the muscles of the chest wall. If a breast tumor was found to have invaded the chest wall, a section of the ribs might be taken as well. The radical mastectomy was a disfiguring operation and might even impair arm movement if there was swelling or nerve damage, but the goal of performing a lifesaving operation took precedence.

A similar philosophy was employed in treating prostate cancer, with the radical perineal prostatectomy to remove a prostate tumor and accompanying lymph nodes in entirety. Concerns over loss of sexual function and continence took a back seat to the need to take one's best shot in the initial surgery to prevent recurrence or spread.

It would be decades before further advances in radiation therapy and chemotherapy allowed surgeons to start to back away from the radical surgical excision of tumors. When rescue therapies such as radiation and chemotherapy became available, surgeons could take a more conservative approach to tumor excision. Radical surgical excisions, however, are still performed today for recurrent pelvic genitourinary or gastrointestinal tumors when all else fails.

Radiation, first discovered around the early 1900s, is generally used to treat a local recurrence of a tumor, to treat a tumor that is not surgically accessible, or to prevent a local recurrence prophylactically. It works by damaging the DNA of rapidly dividing cells, like cancer cells, that are typically growing faster than normal cells, but radiation can also damage normal tissue that may be in the path of an X-ray beam.

Early challenges with radiation therapy included treating tumors deep inside body cavities without burning the skin, and discovering how to focus an X-ray beam on a specific target so that tissues adjacent to a tumor would not be injured. Radiation could be lifesaving, but complications, particularly in terms of late side effects from deep tissue and organ scarring that could worsen over years, could be substantial. It was not unusual, for example, for a patient with prostate cancer who was treated with radiation therapy in the 1960s to suffer substantial damage to organs left behind—the bladder or rectum—that would require removal later, in the 1980s or 1990s. This was because one of the side effects of radiation treatment was inadvertent damage to surrounding blood vessels. Over time these scarred blood vessels would wither away and the surrounding tissues would deteriorate and fall apart. In some cases, the complications of radiation therapy could be fatal.

When President Richard M. Nixon declared war on cancer in 1971, it was with the hope that in marshaling government resources, as was done to split the atom and to put a man on the moon, a cure for cancer would quickly be found. Cancer doctors toiling in the trenches of patient care, however, knew better. While the ravages of cancer were well known then, little was known about how cancer destroyed bodies. Cancer was, in effect, a black box.

"We knew that there were tumors, and we knew that very toxic chemicals could cure some childhood leukemias, or at least put them into remission," Dr. Harold Varmus, a Nobel Prize winner and director of the National Cancer Institute, later recalled.[3] But not a whole lot else was known about cancer.

His admission was as sobering as it was truthful.

There wasn't much optimism about finding a cure for a disease when no one understood what caused it in the first place. Confounding the problem was that cancer was not just one disease. Depending on the organ of origin, cancer could take a myriad of paths that all too often led to a single destination — death. Cancer was, in effect, a hundred different diseases capable of manifesting itself slightly differently in each human host based on his or her own distinct genetic composition.

Since the 1970s, the National Cancer Institute has spent $90 billion on research and treatment. More than 1.2 million Americans develop cancer every year.[4] Cancer is the leading cause of death in individuals under the age of eighty-five and the second cause of death in all age groups. One in five persons in the United States die from cancer every year. Lung and prostate cancer are the top causes of cancer deaths for men, with lung and breast cancers leading for women.

There is no question that major advances in early detection and treatment have been achieved since the war was declared.[5] Death rates for some cancers — breast, lung, prostate, and colorectal cancers — have declined, and overall survival has increased from 50 to 64 percent. There is hope that a new generation of chemotherapeutic drugs that specifically target cancer cells and leave normal cells untouched will cause fewer devastating side effects. We understand more about how cancer does its damage today — that it acts through DNA changes that drive the uncontrolled growth of cancer cells.

For all the measurable progress in individual battles, however, it is an undeniable fact that, forty years into the fight, there's no end in sight for the war on cancer.

By the time the war on cancer was first declared, Dr. Sidney Farber had already been fighting it for almost thirty years. He began his work with cancer patients in 1947, treating a group of childhood leukemia patients that most doctors had given up on because their prospects were so dim. Before taking up childhood cancer, Farber, a pathologist by training, had been working in the basement of the Children's Hospital Medical Center in Boston. He wasn't involved in direct patient care at all when he first started researching the causes and treatment of childhood leukemia. Leukemia, a malignant proliferation of white cells in a person's bloodstream, had a particularly poor prognosis in 1947 because there was no imaginable treatment for a cancer that had invaded a person's bloodstream. It couldn't be cut out in a radical fashion, nor could it be irradiated. Effective cancer fighting drugs had not yet been discovered. Without treatment every child with leukemia faced certain death.

Acute lymphoblastic leukemia (ALL), the most common leukemia of childhood, was particularly frustrating for pediatricians to treat in the 1940s. The uniformly fatal disease could kill a child in a matter of days from the time the characteristic bruising and malaise appeared. The scientific community was pessimistic that a cure would ever be found and was reluctant to devote significant resources to researching leukemia because it appeared so hopeless.[6]

ALL had been discovered almost a century earlier, but there was still little understanding of what caused leukemia. All that was known was that white blood cells produced by the bone marrow proliferated wildly, jamming the bloodstream and, in extreme cases, making the blood appear white rather than red. A normal white blood cell count is 5,000 to 10,000. A leukemia patient's white blood cell count could be 50,000 to 100,000.

In the 1940s, many of the diagnostic tools at our disposal today, such as CT scans and MRIs, did not exist, making the measurement of treatment response in cancer patients difficult without performing an operation before and after treatment. With leukemia, however, treatment response could be monitored by measuring the white blood cell count. If the white blood cell count fell to normal, the disease was in remission. If it started to rise again, the treatment was failing.

A successful treatment for anemia had just been discovered using vitamin B12 and folate injections, both important precursors to DNA formation. Farber, taking a virtual shot in the dark, initially treated a group of patients with folic acid. But instead of stopping the leukemia, folic acid jump-started the disease, causing white blood cell counts to surge.[7] This trial ended in disaster, as the treatment appeared to accelerate white blood cell production and hasten death. Farber was chastised by his colleagues and discouraged from further experimentation.

This monumental failure, however, led to some surprising discoveries. Some tumors showed first accelerated growth followed by regression that might have been related to a secondary folic acid deficiency as the tumors outgrew their blood supply. If there were a drug that could block the action of folic acid on the DNA, a folic acid antagonist, this might slow or possibly even stop the

unchecked flood of white blood cells into the bloodstream. Farber knew of no such drug, but he contacted a colleague, Dr. Yel-
lapragada SubbaRow at the Lederle Laboratories in Pearl River,
New York, who, it turned out, had been developing a class of
drugs with these characteristics. He sent several vials of one of
them, aminopterin, to Farber.

When the drug arrived, Farber rounded up another group of
children with leukemia and began to inject them with the experimental drug aminopterin. There had been no prior animal studies
with the drug. Farber had no knowledge of potential side effects
and could only guess at the dose, but the hallways of his tiny clinic
space were crowded with leukemia patients, all of whom were
facing certain death without treatment. Parents, desperate for
something to slow the progression of the uniformly fatal disease,
put their faith in the one person who had something more than a
prayer to offer.

Farber's initial aminopterin clinical trial was viewed as a success when ten of sixteen children achieved temporary remis-
sions. When Farber published these promising results in the *New
England Journal of Medicine* (1948), however, they were not em-
braced by the scientific community and hailed as the next great
thing in cancer treatment. We can only guess at the reasons why,
but Farber, who had plunged into the world of research with little prior expertise, was viewed as an outsider. Instead of tinkering
in the lab for months to years, trying to understand how a drug
might work and all the potential variations and side effects, he
skipped a few steps and jumped into treating patients. This approach, viewed as reckless by mainstream medicine, was bound
to ruffle the feathers of researchers who had been toiling for years
making only incremental moves that had yielded no promising
treatments and no results even close to the responses Farber had
demonstrated.[8]

Farber, however, was not deterred. He had the firm belief
that cancer could, and would, one day be cured with drug ther-

apy. He continued to push on, experimenting with various combinations of drugs. Unable to secure funding for pediatric cancer research from recognized scientific bodies, he raised his own in record-breaking fashion, enlisting the help of social clubs, Hollywood, and the Boston Red Sox. He took his cause from Hollywood to Congress and the public. The treatment of ALL is today viewed as one of the most successfully treated cancers ever, transforming a disease that was uniformly fatal to one with an 80 percent cure rate, largely because one man dared to go against the grain of what was then considered the conventional wisdom for developing new therapies.

Farber's initial breakthrough with folic acid antagonists led to the development of other drugs to arrest the progression of cancer cells and eventually to using combinations of chemotherapeutic agents, so prevalent and successful today. Aminopterin was eventually replaced with Methotrexate, a less toxic folic acid inhibitor now widely used in the treatment of leukemia, lymphoma, breast cancer, and many other malignancies.

Farber is considered the father of the modern era of chemotherapy, in itself a landmark achievement, but his accomplishments embodied so much more.[9] He is recognized for promoting the concept of locating all cancer patients on a single floor in the hospital so that clinical expertise in treating them could be concentrated in one location. This was important for fostering the skills of nurses, social workers, and other personnel who work with cancer patients and for instituting protocols for specialized cancer care. He later founded one of the first comprehensive pediatric oncology treatment centers, the Children's Cancer Research Foundation, which later became the Dana-Farber Cancer Institute.

About a decade into the war on cancer, I met my first cancer patient, a forty-something housewife with short red hair, a sharp wit, and children about my age. She had lost aunts, uncles, and her mother to colon cancer, and she knew that one day her colon would end up like theirs, coiled and lifeless in a deep stainless steel pan on the back table in an operating room. An orderly in crisp laundered scrubs would deliver it to the pathology lab, where the tumor would be sectioned and examined. The level of invasion through the layers of the colonic wall would be measured, the number of involved lymph nodes counted, and a survival prediction made.

Whereas today a fifteen-minute colonoscopy can pluck out polyps before they have graduated to malignancies, in 1980 "early" detection meant finding a tumor the size of a small anthill outlined on a barium enema. Diagnosing cancer at that stage wouldn't guarantee a cure, but it might tilt the odds in a patient's favor, catching the cancer before it spread. My patient had faithfully swallowed bottles of liquid laxative, taken off from work, and spent entire mornings half clothed in the radiology department, once a year, year after year, for the uncomfortable test — every year except for one. My patient blamed herself when her cancer was diagnosed at an advanced stage, the year she skipped the barium enema. Before she even knew it was there, it had breached the colonic wall, flowed piecemeal through the portal vein, and seeded her liver.

The only effective treatment at that time was the knife, and the cure rate was low. Chemotherapy for metastatic colon cancer was like holy water, something sprinkled around for good measure with little calculable effect. Crude poisons were infused into my patient's bloodstream with the hope they would kill the bad cells and leave the good ones behind.

Even after I read about the cell cycle and about how cancer cells grew faster than normal ones, I was pretty sure the chemo couldn't tell one from the other. I watched how oncologists nudged these patients closer and closer to death, calculating how much more they could stand before the immune system was overrun like an infantry's front line. And when it was, the patients went fast, succumbing to infection in a matter of days or hours.

There was a mythology to this disease, cancer, and people would try anything to stop it, even things that didn't work, even things that could kill them.

At that early stage when I was schooled in the science of medicine but still new to the practice, I clung to the naive expectation that the copper-colored toxins infusing into my patient's veins would save her life or at least give her more time, that everything she had been through—losing her hair and her strength, shaking chills and isolation—would be worth it. But three months later, she was back in the hospital. The cancer that had plowed her liver was now sprouting in her brain, and within weeks it would kill her.

I had entered medical school contemplating a future as an oncologist, intrigued by the challenge of treating the untreatable, but after that rotation I gave it up. I was not gifted with the ability to look into the eyes of one dying patient after another, handing out false hope.

Now we were planning a second-look operation, an exploration of an area of Rachel's body where the unwieldy tumor had been biopsied a few months earlier. We would be reopening a small incision on her back to explore a questionable area noticed on CT scan.

"It's only as big as a pea now," her mother said excitedly, referring to the tumor's shrunken mass now visible only on CT scan. "Isn't that great? And the cancer cells might all be gone by now."

"Yes, it's good news," I said. What this news meant for the future, however, was still uncertain. Rachel had as serious a tumor as a child can have. It was encouraging that this was the only remaining sign of tumor, possibly nothing but a residual scar now, but how long it would remain dormant was something no one could predict.

A cancer prognosis is determined by statistics, a crude measure of predicted survival expressed as a percentage. No one knows where any individual patient will fall on the bell curve. Every statistic, however, is only an average, a gross compilation of some who do really well, some who make out okay, and some who do poorly. I've never really relished the part of the job where you have to try to explain the scary details behind the numbers. Such analysis seems too technical, too cold, to apply to a living, breathing person, a person who means the world to her mother.

Childhood cancer patients face at least two battles. The first and most imminent is the battle to cure the cancer that will take months to years before the words "cure" will ever be uttered. There is a second battle, however, that must be waged over the course of survivors' remaining lifetimes — dealing with the late effects of the initial treatment that saved their lives. Ninety percent of pediatric cancer patients are expected to survive their initial cancer diagnosis, compared to 60 percent of adults; but even after a five-year disease-free interval, designating early cure, childhood cancer patients face a 10 percent increase in mortality compared to a comparable population of patients who did not have cancer.[10] The most common cause of death, occurring in 67 percent, is a recurrence of the original cancer. But there is also a substantial (19 percent) risk that a new cancer will spring to life, a secondary effect of undergoing prior radiation or chemotherapy, both of which may instigate the formation of new cancers as well as curing the original. Breast cancers, for example, may develop after chest irradiation for malignant diseases such as Hodgkin's disease or sarcomas.

In addition to the risk of forming a new cancer, a recent study found that there was also a high rate of chronic disease (up to 73 percent) in childhood cancer survivors even up to thirty years after diagnosis. Radiation and chemotherapy can leave heavy footprints on vital organs. Up to 8 percent of survivors suffer heart dysfunction, most notably from Adriamycin. Up to 9 percent of patients who have had their lungs irradiated develop chronic pulmonary disease such as fibrosis, or scarring within the lungs. Survivors may develop kidney disease, become infertile, and develop cognitive disorders.

Childhood cancer survivors are saddled with the ultimate pre-existing condition and have had difficulty obtaining insurance coverage. With the Affordable Care Act, this burden will hopefully be eased, as denying coverage based on prior health history is no longer permitted.[11]

Survivorship clinics, a relatively new phenomenon, are becoming more prevalent so that oncologists can survey the 1 out of 900 people between the ages of sixteen and forty-four who are survivors of childhood cancer for side effects of cancer treatment. Patients treated in the 1970s and 1980s, when treatment methods were still being refined, are at the greatest risk for chronic health problems. The incidence of such conditions does not diminish over time, as one might expect. Instead, it increases as a person ages.[12] Because of the lifelong risk of side effects and secondary malignancies associated with treatment to cure a child's cancer, ongoing research studies continue to evaluate and refine therapies to minimize these effects.

At Rachel's second operation, about six months after her first, I am peering through magnified lenses looking for the "pea." I have sent several specimens to the pathologist. The first two are negative. He can't find tumor cells in either one. I don't know whether to be relieved that I can't find any disease or concerned because I might be overlooking it.

The next stage of Rachel's treatment, an extended course of radiation, depends on finding out whether there are any viable tumor cells remaining. If there is nothing there to find, she might skip further treatment altogether. But if I miss something that is there, and her treatment is cut short, the disease could return and end her life. Finally, on the verge of giving up, I find a slightly suspicious, thickened edge of muscle. I carve around its indistinct borders and send a third specimen.

The pathologist calls into the operating room. "You found it," he said. "There are definite tumor cells in this last specimen."

After closing, I walk up to the waiting room, anticipating that Rachel's mother will be upset with the news, the way she was after the first operation when she learned of the diagnosis. On my way in, I look around for a box of tissues for the inevitable eruption of tears. I sit down next to her and explain where we took the biopsies and how we sent each one to the pathologist for a frozen section examination. I dance around the news until I can't any more, and finally I just say it. *The last mass we removed, although small, contained active tumor cells.*

"Isn't that great?" she says. "It was so small you could hardly find it, and now that it's out she's disease free for the first time in six months."

Surprised by her response, I stop and think. Could she be right? Is this news worth celebrating?

Inside my head, a fear of the great unknown is colliding with this mother's unrestrained expression of joy. There is still the possibility that microscopic deposits of malignant cells are lurking somewhere else in the muscle, lymph nodes, virtually anywhere in Rachel's small body. They might band together some day, rise up, grow wildly out of control, and put an end to her life.

I know her mother knows that same thing. She knows it is for exactly this reason that her daughter has gone through months of operations, chemotherapy, infections, hair loss, and tears. But she has shown me something that is so easy to forget when you are caught up in the minutiae of diseases and treatment, of being a doctor and not a mother. For this moment, neither the past nor the future matters. What matters is today and, for today, the news is worth celebrating.

tiny tools for tiny bodies

Without looking up I extend my hand to the side and slightly behind me, expecting to feel the featherweight of the neonatal chest retractor drop lightly into my palm. Instead, something more like a shovel hits — an adult Balfour retractor, about ten by six inches across, twice the baby's size and big enough to crush this tiny birdlike creature.

The retractor that I now hold in my hands is something general surgeons shoehorn into the belly of adults to hold the abdominal wall out of the way. I hand it back. I tell the scrub nurse this isn't the right one. Not even close. I describe the one we need, the neonatal chest retractor, the smallest one made.

At this point, one would think a solution would be readily at hand, perhaps as simple as calling the supply room and swapping out the big abdominal retractor for the tiny chest retractor. But we are not in the main operating room, where all the supplies are kept. We are upstairs working in the NICU in a procedure room about the size of a janitor's closet because the baby is too unstable to make the trip downstairs to the operating room.

There are no surplus supplies up here, only what the nurses brought up to begin with. Even if someone runs down a flight of stairs to the operating room central supply and rifles through every bin that contains chest or neonatal equipment at a frenetic pace, it will take too long to find the retractor we need.

We can't leave a 500-gram (just over a pound) preemie on his side for long. His waterlogged lungs are barely inflating now. The pulse oximeter (oxygen monitor) at the head of the bed shows his oxygen level pivoting between low and dangerously low even on 100 percent oxygen. The baby, teetering on the brink of cardio-vascular collapse, could dive into the danger zone any minute and fail to resurface.

Our patient, one of the smallest humans alive, is under the drapes, turned on his side, and we have just started opening his chest, in-cising the muscle between his matchstick ribs. We have about a quarter inch opening, and now we need the neonatal chest retrac-tor, a two-by-one-inch metal rib spreader with two blunt blades made to be pushed gently into the opening. Once the retractor is inserted, we will rotate the hand crank that gently pulls the open-ing apart and holds it open while we're working in an opening the size of a domino.

Our mission is to ligate the ductus arteriosus, a blood vessel that, during gestation, allows most of a fetus's circulation, oxy-genated by his mother, to bypass his fluid-filled lungs and flow directly into his aorta. Normally the duct closes within the first twelve to twenty-four hours after birth, but in some premature infants the duct persists and becomes as large as the aorta, the main blood vessel in the body. The increased flow of blood to the lungs causes respiratory distress, and the decreased flow through the aorta leads to kidney failure and possible intestinal inflamma-tion. Many times a duct will close with medication alone, but if it doesn't, a surgeon will have to close it with a clip.

The clips come in three sizes — small, medium, and large. It was a relief to find them lined up on the Mayo stand, rigid and straight, as if at attention in their white, green, and blue rectangu-lar plastic holders, poised and waiting for the big event.

Before the start of the operation I had inspected the stainless steel clip applier to make sure the tips lined up perfectly when I squeezed them together to compress the clip. If the tips had in-stead scissored past each other like subway cars on parallel tracks, the clip would twist as it closed, and the blood vessel would tear. In the ensuing seconds of terror the baby's entire blood volume could pour out of a flea-sized speck of a hole, flooding the surgical field with a dark swirl of blood. It was a kind of bleeding that wouldn't stop easily, an unwelcome race between control and exsanguination that might incite the flinging of a barrage of clips and hemostats in the direction of a hole they could only wish to close.

I checked the clips. I never dreamed I'd have to check the retractor too.

Every pediatric surgeon knows the disheartening feeling of not having the right size tool to start with or having something that can't be replaced break or fall on the floor. There aren't a lot of extras of anything lying around in size "tiny" to begin with. A missing tool might be in the wrong instrument pack. A broken one might have been sent out for repair. They may have worn out and not been replaced because of a capital equipment budget oversight. Maybe it's not a big deal because something else will do, or maybe the missing tool adds one more degree of difficulty to an already trying situation.

The default size for equipment in hospitals is adult because adults make up the vast majority of patients in most hospitals. Medic Joey Falcone echoed this fact after returning from the war in Afghanistan. "All of my equipment was for adults. Whenever a kid got wounded, I would try to improvise because everything was smaller. Their limbs are smaller. Airways smaller. Smaller organs."[1] Pediatric surgery patients come in a range of ages and sizes, from two-pound premature infants to two-hundred-pound obese adolescents.

To deviate from the default, someone has to go to the trouble to locate an alternative, downsized version, get it approved for purchase, and order it. This isn't going to happen automatically. Someone is going to have to recognize the need and request the right size of even the most mundane items. Even a simple toddler-sized gown with teddy bear appliqués for a child to change into in the preop holding area has to be ordered.

There are other devices besides tools that have to be kept in stock in the operating room. The anesthesiologist needs a breathing tube about the size of the patient's little finger. A child needs a smaller IV catheter. The IV tubing has to be smaller to prevent accidental fluid overdoses. The OR nurse applies a self-sticking grounding pad for the electrocautery, the size determined by patient weight; the little bitty white one is a must-have for the smallest babies, like this one. It measures approximately two by four inches and works for any baby weighing 4.8 pounds or less. The big blue adult pad would have to wrap around the baby's body three times, leaving no bare skin for an incision.

The pediatric operating table is narrower and shorter than the full-sized adult model. When a bed is too wide, the surgeon has to stand too far away from his tiny patient to work on him up close. Even the EKG leads have to be smaller. Adult-sized leads as big as a baby's head are just too big. Before we ever get to the actual equipment to be used to perform the operation, just to get to the starting line, a significant investment must be made and attention paid to all these details.

So what do we do without the chest retractor?

We'll have to use something else to pull the opening apart, like two handheld army-navy tissue retractors hooked around the ribs. They won't work as well. This will mean more hands involved, introducing more movement, more distraction, as we try to focus on the minuscule structures we're working on. We won't be able to see as well, and the makeshift solution will slow us down, but there is no other choice at this exact moment. We can't cancel the procedure with the baby under anesthesia and the chest open, so we're going to do what pediatric surgeons have always done — make it up as we go along using the best tools we have, whether or not they're a perfect fit.

In 1987, Dr. Melvin Smith, a pediatric surgeon in San Antonio, Texas, was consulted on a six-month-old infant born with severe scoliosis and missing seven of twelve ribs. The chest wall does not grow normally in babies born with fused or absent ribs. They are small and misshapen and lack sufficient structural support to allow the lungs to develop. Without treatment the babies' chests slowly collapse, while their spines curve over on themselves like a twisted tree limb. Within weeks to months the infants all become ventilator dependent, and eventually most die from a lack of oxygen.

Shortly after birth the child had been transferred to Houston doctors, who attempted an external brace, but it did not help him. The boy was sent back home to San Antonio with a dismal prognosis.[2]

This debilitating condition, thoracic insufficiency syndrome, affected less than a hundred children a year in the United States. Smith knew of nothing that would help the child, but he hoped that the doctors who repaired spinal deformities, pediatric orthopedic surgeons, might be able to come up with a solution to stabilize the boy's chest wall. He approached first one orthopedic surgeon and then a second. Neither had anything to offer. But the third orthopedic surgeon Smith consulted, Dr. Robert Campbell, had studied engineering before entering medical school and was intrigued by the clinical dilemma. He thought there might be a way to use plates or wires to construct a chest wall. He told Smith he would see what he could come up with and get back to him.

Campbell went home that same night and sketched out a procedure to stabilize the chest wall using tools and materials that he worked with every day. He had to reimagine the use of Kirschner wires, smooth stainless steel pins that were normally used to hold bony fragments together. The pins were usually inserted into the longitudinal axis of a fractured bone. In fashioning a substitute for missing ribs, he would need to position the pins around the child's chest and across the gap. But Campbell worried that if the pins shifted or migrated they could puncture the child's heart or lung on the front side of the chest or erode into his spinal cord at the back, where the ribs joined the spine.

To make the procedure safer, Campbell proposed turning the pins 90 degrees so that they would be inserted vertically rather than horizontally to form a bridge over the gap where the chest wall had failed to form. The next step was to twist the wires around the surrounding ribs to hold them in place.[3] The procedure had never been attempted. No one knew whether it would work or what the possible complications might be, but there were no other alternatives to save a child who would eventually suffocate if nothing was done.

New inventions begin with an idea inspired by a need. Bob Kearns was driving through the streets of Detroit in 1962 when a light rain began. Windshield wipers at that time had two settings— low and high. When it was only drizzling outside, the wipers screeched across the windshield, smearing the glass.[4] Straining to see through an eye that had been injured by a champagne cork on his wedding night, and frustrated by a worn pair of wipers, an idea flickered into Kearns's consciousness. *Why couldn't a windshield wiper work more like the blink of an eyelid, moving intermittently rather than constantly back and forth?*

That one question became the incentive for Kearns's invention. A mechanical engineer studying for his PhD at the time, he worked on the project at home on the weekends. He created an intermittent wiper using electronics to vary the timing of the wiper movement. At one point he even installed an aquarium in his basement and filled it with a mixture of oil, sawdust, and water to test his intermittent wipers. Eventually he perfected his model and it was adopted throughout the industry.[5]

An inventor's "flash of genius," the moment when a unique solution suddenly appears like a divine apparition, has formed the basis for many life-changing inventions. New medical devices tend to come about in this same way. Almost always, the need that inspires them is that of a patient, usually one in particularly dire straits. In this case the inventions are not just life changing but also lifesaving.

Starting in high school in the 1940s, Tom Fogarty worked as a scrub tech at Good Samaritan Hospital in Cincinnati, Ohio. Time after time, he watched patients with blood clots in their arms or legs come through the operating room, and the results were not good. Blood clots blocked the flow of blood through the length of an extremity. If an artery was blocked for longer than six hours, the viability of a patient's limb would be jeopardized. To make matters worse, the blood clots tended to recur, and most patients required multiple operations. Half of them died and 50 percent of those who survived needed amputations.

The operation to remove a blood clot involved opening up the entire length of an artery, a time-consuming process that required a long incision and incurred substantial blood loss.[6] Fogarty wondered if there could be a better way. With the support of a surgeon who became his mentor, he eventually made it to medical school, where he started tinkering and came up with a device that would allow a surgeon to access a blood clot from a distance.[7]

"I cut the baby finger off of a surgical glove and tied that onto the end of a catheter with fly-tying techniques I learned as a boy," Fogarty later recalled.[8]

He used the finger of the glove like a balloon. When empty and flat it could be inserted into an artery, and threaded past the site of a blood clot. Once past the clot it could be filled with saline through a channel in the catheter and then pulled back out, fishing out the clot on the way and opening up the blood vessel so that blood could again travel through the artery.

Fogarty later explained his flash of genius moment when the idea for the balloon catheter came to him. "It was like you see in a cartoon," he said. "It was like a bomb goes off in your mind."[9]

He started making the catheters himself and, in 1961, gave one to a surgeon he scrubbed for who used it himself in the operating room and passed it around to his colleagues to try. The FDA had not yet started regulating medical devices, and all Fogarty needed was the approval of the chief of surgery at the hospital. It took only six weeks from the time Fogarty first produced the device to the time a surgeon used one on a patient.

Fogarty's device was entirely new and showed great promise, but at first he couldn't get anyone to manufacture his catheter to remove blood clots. The companies he approached thought a medical student couldn't possibly know what he was doing, but Fogarty kept trying. With the assistance of a cardiovascular surgeon, Fogarty made contact with Edwards Life Science, a company willing to take a chance that his balloon catheter would become a successful product that surgeons would adopt into practice.

Fogarty's technique for removing blood clots became the standard of care because his new procedure posed less risk to the patient, shortened the time for the operation, and worked. Today the Fogarty catheter, or some variation, is stocked in every hospital operating room and radiology department in America and many foreign countries. It is used in approximately 300,000 operations a year and has saved the lives of millions of patients.

Everyone thinks of inventors as being creative, out-of-the-box thinkers, and Fogarty certainly fit the mold, but when asked the key to success, he said it was "persistence to the point of obnoxiousness."[10] Every time a physician inventor trots out something new, he butts heads with the status quo — the ingrained practice patterns of physicians and their extreme aversion to change. Inventors must be tenacious, self-confident, and able to persevere through failure to see their idea actually gain traction in medical practice.

"If there's one lesson I've learned it's to never give up," Fogarty said.[11]

His body of work is testimony to the fact that he didn't. Fogarty went on to become the founder or cofounder of thirty-three companies and acquired over one hundred patents. Known as the "Edison of Medicine," he is credited for starting the movement toward minimally invasive procedures by developing techniques that can be performed through smaller incisions. He was a pioneer in cardiac angioplasty, a technique that supplanted the need for open-heart surgery to remove a clot from a blood vessel in the heart.[12] In 2007 he founded the Fogarty Institute for Innovation, where he mentors and trains medical device inventors, including high school and college students interested in a career in medicine or medical innovation.[13]

When Smith and Campbell operated on the infant with thoracic insufficiency syndrome, they found, as expected, a sunken chest wall rimmed by bent and undersized ribs. They measured and cut the pins to fit the area to be reconstructed. Campbell then used a set of sterile vise grips to twist the end of three pins around the ribs on either side of the chest wall defect. Smith inserted a sheet of Silastic underneath the pins to protect the lung and add support to the repair. Then they closed.

When they looked at the postoperative chest X-ray, the surgeons discovered that the artificial chest wall they had created not only stabilized the child's lung function but also straightened the curvature that had developed in his spine, an unexpected by-product of stabilizing the chest wall. Within a week the infant was weaned off the ventilator for the first time in his life.

As the child's condition improved, the surgeons realized that their young patient would eventually outgrow the chest wall they had created. With the goal of avoiding the need to perform a major operation every few years to replace the pins, Campbell set out to create a new chest wall prosthesis that was not only easy to implant but could be serially adjusted with only a minor operation. Campbell envisioned a device that would work like a curtain rod, a bar that could be expanded periodically to stretch across the widening defect as the child grew. He chose titanium as the material, not only because it was lightweight but also because it was biocompatible and would not interfere with future MRIs.

Having an idea is just the beginning of the long road to bringing a new medical device to the market. The idea must be translated into a working prototype, a step that may require collaborating with an engineer. Assuming that the device is unique, that there is room in the patent space for this new concept, the inventors must file for a patent to protect their commercial rights. Then the device has to be tested in the laboratory to assess its efficacy and safety. The experimental results may indicate that the device needs to be modified. This will mean bringing back the engineer and possibly acquiring more experimental data. All of these steps add expense and can swallow huge chunks of time — months, even years — before the product makes it to the clinical market.

Before any implantable devices can be marketed in the United States, the FDA must conduct a premarket review process that generally involves the submission of extensive experimental data regarding the safety and effectiveness of the device.[14] This is a time-consuming and costly step. The FDA review may indicate that further testing is required in greater numbers or that the device must be modified, both of which will add to the project's cost. The FDA may require more data, and possibly even clinical trials in humans, before a device is approved for sale.

The expenses to achieve all these steps may total from several hundred thousand dollars to over a million depending on the complexity of the device and its intended purpose, and they are all incurred before one dime of revenue is generated from the sale of the device. Very few devices make it very far without venture capitalists, independent investors who will examine an inventor's track record, expertise, and experimental design with a magnifying glass before they dump their cash into a project.

It is easy to see why the vast majority of medical products that enter clinical trials ultimately fail to reach the market.[15] An inventor could easily run out of money, hit a regulatory snag, or discover a competing product that he cannot design around. Many inventions are abandoned after extensive investment that is never recouped.

"Inventing it turned out to be the easy part," Campbell later said about the titanium rib.[16] Finding a company to manufacture a totally new device for use in only one patient would turn out to be more difficult. He approached several orthopedic device manufacturers and was eventually referred to Techmedica, a custom prosthesis company that made artificial joints.[17] By the time Campbell first met with the company, it had been a year since he and Smith had first operated on the boy. Their patient had begun to catch up on his growth and was gaining weight, but his spine was starting to curve again. The return of his scoliosis indicated he would soon need more chest support.

In the meeting with Techmedica the CEO asked Campbell how many patients a year would need the artificial ribs. Campbell's best guess at the time was that it would only be a handful of patients a year, not enough to make the project profitable to Techmedica. The CEO could sense Campbell's desperation but also his dedication. Campbell wasn't making any money off the deal either. He was just trying to find someone to make a device to treat a needy little boy. Techmedica agreed to manufacture the titanium ribs even though the company would likely lose money on the project. All the CEO asked in return was some favorable publicity if it turned out that the device worked.

Two years after his first surgery, the boy was the recipient of the first vertical expandable prosthetic titanium rib (VEPTR). The VEPTR is an adjustable titanium rod that expands to allow for growth, is curved like a ribcage to allow more volume for the lung, and has hooks on either end that attach to the ribs. The boy did well after the second operation and had the rod adjusted every six months in a relatively simple procedure performed in outpatient surgery. Eventually his bones matured when he was in his late teens and the regular rib adjustments were no longer necessary.[18]

After using the device successfully on selective patients under the custom medical device exception, the surgeons realized that the next step was to seek FDA approval so the VEPTR could become widely available to those in need. As part of the FDA application process they would need experimental data, so in the mid-1990s Campbell and Smith initiated a clinical trial to test the titanium rib. The trial included patients from six other children's hospitals. Because the condition was rare, it took years to accumulate a sufficient number of patients to satisfy the FDA. In 2004, seventeen years and three hundred operations after the first titanium rib was implanted, the device was finally approved.

Not only was the VEPTR a huge clinical success (families across the country lined up for Campbell to operate on them); it also became the poster child for how pediatric medical devices get bogged down in the regulatory process. Because children are a smaller percentage of the population, acquiring sufficient numbers to satisfy the FDA can cause unreasonable delays in what is already a cumbersome approval process. Campbell testified before Congress in 2007 citing his difficulties obtaining FDA approval and pointing out that it can take up to a decade longer for a pediatric device to be approved than one for adults.[19]

In this ultra-high-tech, postmillennial, supercomputing world of ours, it seems counterintuitive that medical devices tailored to fit a pediatric patient are still lacking, but that is indeed the case. In 2011 the FDA confirmed that the development of medical devices for children still lagged five to ten years behind the adult market.[20] This is not surprising when one considers that it can be just as costly to develop a pediatric medical device as it is to develop one for adults, but the available market is considerably smaller. While the market for pediatric devices varies according to the individual disease process a device is intended to treat, the overall percentage of the US population aged seventeen and under is currently only 24 percent and dropping—or roughly a third of the adult market.[21] Children with unusual or rare conditions represent just a sliver of that number. No matter how brilliant a potential medical product might be, it will bump up against the profitability question when it comes time to sell the idea to a medical device manufacturer. Very few companies can afford to make devices that lose money.

There are other factors unique to pediatrics that further complicate the pediatric medical device landscape. Besides the fact that pediatric patients are smaller and devices must be downsized to fit, the pediatric population is, at a minimum, four distinct subpopulations: neonates, infants, children, and adolescents. When a medical device company manufactures a pediatric product, it needs to be produced in at least four sizes and possibly more.

Children's bodies are proportioned differently from adults. These proportions and the child's size change over time, characteristics that must be taken into account in product design. The physiology, the growth rate, the activity level, and many bodily functions are distinctly different from those of adults. For example, not only are a child's bones smaller than an adult's; they are also softer, and they have growth plates on either end that are uniquely susceptible to injury. A company manufacturing an orthopedic device to be used in children would have to take all these characteristics into account. A young child may have to undergo multiple operations to change out a device that he has outgrown, or a device that has worn out over years of use. The failure rate of cardiac defibrillators in children, for example, is 20–25 percent, while adult defibrillators hardly ever fail.[22]

Clinical trials of new devices in children can be problematic because of safety concerns. Parents may be understandably reluctant to consent to an experimental device. This can make it

difficult for a company to recruit enough children to enroll in
a clinical trial, especially if a particular condition for which the
device is intended is uncommon.[23] Recently the FDA has waived
some fees for pediatric medical devices being considered under
the humanitarian device exemption, hoping to disencumber the
process of pediatric medical device approval. While it is still too
early to assess the effects of these new initiatives, the FDA continues to study the disparate impact of the FDA approval process on
the pediatric market and seems willing to make further changes
to speed the approval of pediatric medical devices.

In the meantime, while pediatric surgeons and other pediatric
subspecialists wait for the devices they need, they continue to improvise and adapt equipment made for adults to meet the needs
of their smaller patients. These solutions are not optimal and pose
their own sets of hazards, as illustrated by the case of a child who
at a young age needed an artificial mitral valve, a valve that controls the flow of blood between the left atrium and the left ventri-
cle. The only available valve, an adult mechanical valve, was too
large to fit in the proper position and had to be implanted above
the anatomically correct position in the heart. With less than
ideal placement, the child developed heart failure and required
a heart transplant to survive, an unlikely scenario if the valve had
been positioned properly.[24]

Unfortunately, there are many diseases and conditions so rare
that the cost of research and development for products to diagnose and treat them outweighs the monetary return on investment. In light of this fact, the FDA has created the Office of
Orphan Products Development to encourage the development
of these products.[25] Two specific programs address these needs.
The Orphan Drug program incentivizes the development of drugs
that would be applicable to fewer than 200,000 patients per year
in the United States, and the Humanitarian Use Device Program

(HUD) subsidizes the development of medical devices or products that fewer than 4,000 patients per year could use.

In 2007 Congress passed the Pediatric Medical Device Safety and Improvement Act, authorizing the FDA to offer grants to assist in funding the development of pediatric devices.[26] The Pediatric Device Consortia Grants Program funds nonprofit consortiums of physicians, engineers, and scientists to stimulate the development of pediatric medical devices. The FDA has dispensed $11 million in grants to nonprofit pediatric medical device consortiums. In theory, if Campbell and Smith were proposing the titanium rib today, they would have access to advisers experienced in regulatory requirements, business development, intellectual property, engineering, laboratory/animal testing, grant writing, and clinical trial design who would help streamline the process of bringing the titanium rib to the market.[27]

One new device that may benefit from the FDA's pediatric medical device initiative is the Magnetic Mini Mover (3MP), aimed at restoring a normal chest contour to children born with pectus excavatum, or sunken chest deformity.[28] This deformity not only affects body image but can also compromise heart and lung function and decrease exercise tolerance. Currently, to repair pectus excavatum requires a major operation that involves either removing deformed cartilage from ribs on both sides of the sternum or inserting a bar under the breastbone (sternum) and pushing it outward. These operations, which surgeons describe as "brutal," require hospitalizations of up to a week just to treat the postoperative pain.

In a new approach devised by surgeons, engineers, and orthotics experts, a round magnet is screwed into the sternum in an outpatient procedure. The chest is gradually drawn forward by another magnet inserted into a chest protector that the patient wears. The assembled product resembles the electromagnetic arc reactor that keeps Iron Man's heart beating. Gradually repositioning the rib cartilages is similar to moving the teeth with orthodontic braces and much less painful than the all-at-once approach currently practiced.

Like any new implantable device, the 3MP has required extensive testing not only to prove it works but also to be sure it is safe. During the initial phase of animal and/or human use, observations are made that lead to modifications. In the end there is only so much the FDA can do to speed the process, as all phases of development and patient enrollment in FDA trials takes time.

The first 3MP was implanted into a fourteen-year-old boy in 2007, part of the first FDA trial, reported in 2010. Ultimately, ten patients were enrolled and the 3MP was found to be safe and cost effective.[29] The current phase III trial, in progress since 2011, is expected to conclude in 2016, after which, if the device is proven safe and effective, one would expect it to be commercially available. That is a nine-year lag from first insertion to widespread availability. In the meantime more data will be accumulated and possibly more modifications made that may or may not require additional testing. If the 3MP is proven to be effective over the long term, it will provide a less invasive, less painful, less costly treatment option for pectus excavatum than the current operations.

Three-dimensional (3-D) printing technology is another advance that will bring down the cost of customizing a medical device prototype to the size of an individual patient. A 3-D printer uses a digital computer file to print out a tangible object by stacking layers of materials such as metal, plastic, or nylon.[30] Almost any geometrical shape imaginable can be produced. This is exactly the type of technology that might help a two-year-old who needs a smaller mitral valve. Theoretically, the design of the existing adult-sized valve could be laser scanned with a computer software program. The design would then be downsized using the same program and the new valve printed out from a composite of biocompatible material. 3-D printing will eliminate the need for traditional molds, tools, and dies currently used to produce different-shaped products. Producing smaller products will no longer add overhead to the manufacturing process.

Miniaturization of surgical tools, in general, is on a hot streak, as technology has finally caught up with the need for smaller instruments. For example, there are now cameras small enough to see into salivary gland ducts, and tools to match that can clear out blockages.[31] A team at Johns Hopkins has created new microscopically small biopsy tools as small as a speck of dust.[32] These can be deployed into the gastrointestinal tract through the mouth and directed to obtain a piece of tissue at a specific location. Children stand to benefit from this trend of producing smaller and smaller tools because once they are available they can be adapted for pediatric use.

The days when pediatric surgeons had to operate with one hand tied behind their backs struggling with adult-sized instruments and devices, improvising and downsizing just to get something to work or fit, are coming to a close. In the near future, operating on a baby will no longer be fraught with mismatched tools and devices that have to be coaxed into awkward positions in miniature body cavities. Tiny tools that fit tiny bodies will at last be feasible and affordable.

10 lessons

"Have you ever done anything to kill a kid?" Dr. R. asked me shortly after I had begun training with him.

He was a slightly stooped, gray-haired man with bushy, unruly eyebrows. The bow tie he wore signaled that he was an absolute expert on every topic in surgery. He rocked back and forth on the balls of his wingtips and looked me in the eye. He was dead serious.

"No, sir. Not that I'm aware of," I answered.

"Well, then, you're a very lucky person," he said. "Sooner or later you will."

Dr. R. and I rounded together daily. Like a pointer tracking the scent of prey, he sniffed out all sorts of things we surgeons-in-training had failed to notice. *Was the nasogastric tube truly in the stomach and suctioning the contents properly? Was there skin redness around the* IV sites, indicating infection? Had I done a complete physical from head to toe to find the source of that low-grade fever? He seemed picky, obsessive, even obnoxious at times. His incessant questions grated on my nerves, but they did serve a purpose.

Dr. R. had been in the pediatric surgery business long enough to understand that the hospital was a dangerous place. From the moment a child changed into his or her teddy bear pajamas and took on the identity of "patient," each person who came in contact with them was just as likely to accidentally hurt them as to help them. This especially applied to us, the surgeons, because with our sharp instruments we stood to do the most damage. If we didn't pay attention to every single detail, no matter how mundane, we were sure to incur a complication.

A medical complication is a secondary condition that arises in the course of treating a patient's primary medical problem, the reason they came to the hospital in the first place. Complications are unexpected. They are not supposed to happen, but they do.

Some complications are unavoidable, like a patient who has an unexpected allergic reaction to a medication and suffers a cardiac arrest. No one could have predicted or prevented the reaction. Other complications might have been prevented before the genie ever got out of bottle. For example, if antibiotics aren't given thirty minutes before the incision is made, a patient could develop an infection at the incision site. The wound infection could be minor and relatively short-lived, or it could spread like a rumor in a middle school, dissolving skin and sutures and requiring multiple drainage procedures to get it under control. At the very least it would annoy the patient, cause needless physical pain, potentially worsen the scar, and result in additional expense and days missed from work or school.

Some but not all complications result from mistakes — in other words, medical error. Certain complications can result from technical mistakes that occur in the operating room, such as tying off a blood vessel that should have been left alone, suturing or cutting too deeply, all of which can damage a nearby structure. Other complications are the result of errors in judgment — performing the wrong operation at the wrong time or choosing the wrong antibiotic to give before an operation. A complication like leaving a sponge or instrument inside a patient falls into a different class altogether. Attorneys refer to this kind of medical error as *res ipsa loquitur*, Latin for "the thing speaks for itself." There is no need to bring in experts to debate whether malpractice has occurred because this type of mistake, in general, is indefensible. By virtue of the event happening, the verdict has already been decided.

Changing the course of a patient after a major complication is like trying to steer the *Titanic* after it has already smashed into the iceberg. From the time disaster strikes, any progress toward discharge from the hospital will be incremental. Nothing humbles a surgeon like watching a patient lose ground day after day from a series of complications. Every extra day that the patient is in the hospital, the surgeon's mistake will be staring him in the face, a reminder of his imperfection.

One of Dr. R.'s favorite things to do when we were operating together was to recite from memory the worst complication that had ever occurred in association with the particular operation we were performing. This might be one of his own mistakes, to which he readily admitted, or it might be somebody else's, too sensational not to share, sotto voce, as if he were leaning across a Formica table in a coffee shop instead of a patient's still, anesthetized body.

For example, if we were taking out the spleen, he would recall the time a surgeon in a distant state had taken out a kidney by accident during a routine splenectomy. This disturbing narrative was not just idle banter. Dr. R. dug out these horror stories to instruct, explaining exactly how such an error could occur, even with the best of surgeons.

"It had to be because of the incision," he related. His insider analysis deduced that the incision must have been too small. There was not enough exposure to get a complete view of the internal organs and their relation to each other. With only a partial view the surgeon had gotten confused.

I was too focused on the spleen we were taking out to absorb his story fully. Or so I thought in the moment. Only later, during other surgeries, did I realize how powerful his telling was—not just the *what* of it, but the *when* of it, the lessons spewing forth under the bright lights of the operating room with tools in hand, in situations eerily similar to that of the ill-fated tales.

To this day, every time I take out a spleen, I feel for the left kidney below. I know exactly where the spleen is and what it looks like. I don't think I've ever even come close to mistaking it for any other organ. But Dr. R.'s horror stories prompt a Pavlovian need for me to perform my ritualistic palpation every time.

Healthcare is riddled with medical errors — errors in diagnosis and treatment, errors in communication, equipment failure that harms a patient. This fact became widely known in 1999 after the Institute of Medicine (IOM) reported that at least 98,000 patients a year died in US hospitals as a result of mistakes, a number equivalent to one jumbo jetliner crashing every day.[1] Surgeons operate on the wrong body part approximately forty times per week. Twenty-five percent of hospitalized patients will be harmed by some kind of mistake.[2]

Most experts agree that medical errors are underestimated because, for the most part, they are voluntarily reported. It can also be difficult to capture accurate data in a system where undesirable outcomes and deaths may have multifactorial causes — that is, the patient's underlying disease contributes to a poor outcome in the face of a medical error. In a more recent study, one in which medical errors were counted by experts reviewing charts, the number of premature deaths in hospitals associated with a preventable harm ballooned dramatically to a range of 210,000 to 420,000 patients per year in the United States.[3] While this number seems staggering (two to four jumbo jetliners per day), leading healthcare safety experts who reviewed the data agreed that this number was entirely feasible.

These shocking statistics inevitably raise the question: *What kind of shop are we running in the medical profession?*

Airlines are cited as a model of how an industry learns from its mistakes. Detailed cockpit checklists and procedures are followed before takeoff to detect potential mechanical problems on the ground. Every time a plane crashes, the National Transportation Safety Board (NTSB) performs an independent investigation, and the findings are widely broadcast within the industry.

Healthcare, however, has been anything but transparent in terms of publicizing mistakes that harm patients and, compared to other high-risk industries, has been slow to develop reactive practices that enhance patient safety. Lawsuits and the fear of tarnishing the reputations of physicians and hospitals have overshadowed the development of a national system to report and collect data on medical mistakes. During the last decade, however, hospitals, doctors, and the federal government have been putting measures in place to grapple with safety issues. The Agency for Healthcare Research and Quality, a division of the Department of Health and Human Services, was born in the aftermath of the alarming IOM report with a mission of improving healthcare quality, efficiency, and effectiveness. Compared to a $27 billion budget for the National Institutes of Health, however, its annual budget is a mere $60 million.

The Joint Commission for Accreditation of Health Care Organizations (JCAHO), a nonprofit that inspects and grades hospital quality, requires that hospitals report all serious adverse events and perform a root cause analysis of why they occurred. Individual hospitals have instituted programs such as computerized mandatory error reporting and preoperative surgical site marking in an attempt to get control of the medical error epidemic. Some hospitals have even taken the step of hiring a safety officer, an individual who investigates the causes of medical errors and leads efforts to prevent them.

Many hospitals now require the preoperative timeout to be performed before every operation, just like in a cockpit before takeoff. During this timeout, the operating room team goes through a checklist: the surgical consent is read aloud, the patient's identity is confirmed, the operation to be performed is confirmed, and any special conditions, such as a medication allergy, are noted. Communication is established among team members, including the surgeon, anesthesiologist, scrub tech, and circulating nurse. This is an attempt to make sure everyone is on the same page before the operation begins, and if they are not, if anyone in the room senses a problem, she is encouraged to speak up and identify the issue.

Every surgeon I know agrees that the timeout is a great idea. Why did it take so long to implement? Some believe the culture of medicine itself may have impeded the adoption of checklists and other team-based protocols that could alleviate the medical error deluge. Physicians have always been the undisputed decision makers regarding the treatment of their patients. No one questioned what the surgeon was going to do in the operating room. Everyone assumed he knew which side of the body to open up and what to do when he got in there.

The same top-down approach once dominated the airline industry, with a pilot functioning as the unquestioned authority-in-chief, but that changed after several high-profile plane crashes in the 1970s in which pilot error was key. After that the aviation industry decided that the existing hierarchy would have to be dismantled to make air travel safer.

The patients filling up that one jumbo jetliner a day (or possibly more) are spread across thousands of hospitals in the United States. Their numbers are diluted in our consciousness, but if all those patients were falling out of the sky at the same time, we wouldn't be able to deny the reality of the tragedy. We can't always prevent patients from dying of diseases, but we should be able to curtail the rampant epidemic of medical errors.

Years after my training with Dr. R., I can almost feel him in the room with me, every time I am even close to making a mistake. Like an arthritic knee that begins to ache as a cold front is blowing in, his words echo in my ears and I start to tense up. I hear them now during what should be a routine case, and I don't even know for sure that something is wrong.

We have finally reached the simple part of the operation. The first two hours were spent working in a newborn's chest, separating a wayward esophagus that had taken a wrong turn and fused with the backside of the trachea. Now we have moved on to inserting a simple feeding tube into the stomach of the premature infant. This is the easy part of the case, the part that you can do in your sleep or with one hand tied behind your back. It is the part that should go smoothly and without incident.

The tube is in. We have filled a balloon that keeps it in place and checked its position in the stomach, and now we are suturing the tube into place, and that's when I see it: a tiny wisp of yellow out of the corner of my eye.

"Did you see that?" I ask the surgeon assisting me.

"What?" he says.

"That yellow stuff. Where did that come from?" The fluid inside the intestinal tract is greenish yellow, a mixture of bile and gastric acid. It would be okay if a little bit had leaked out when we made the hole to put the tube in, but there shouldn't be any leaking out now.

"I didn't see anything," he says.

But then another trace of yellow crosses my visual field, off to the side of where I am working. I pick up a syringe of saline and wash the area. Now all the fluid is clear, like it is supposed to be. Maybe I was just imagining things.

"It all looks good to me," my assistant says. "I think we should close."

My assistant is growing impatient with me. It is a Saturday and he has about a million places he would rather be than in the 80-degree heat of this operating room.

"Okay, just give me a minute," I say. I pick up a syringe, attach it to the end of the tube, and flush it with water. I'm looking to see if the stomach inflates or if the water is leaking out through a hole that shouldn't be there. The water floods up from behind the stomach. Something is wrong.

"Did you see that?" I ask him.

"I think it's leaking around the tube," he says. "Maybe you just need to cinch it down with another stitch."

I put in another suture, wishing, hoping for an easy fix. I'm tired. I was on call the night before and got very little sleep. I want this operation to end too. I pick up the syringe again and test the tube. More saline floods out from somewhere it shouldn't be. This time I'm sure. The saline is not coming from around the tube. There is something wrong. I don't just suspect it now; I feel it, viscerally.

There has to be a leak somewhere. I don't know where it is or how it got there, and we can't tell by looking into the tiny incision we've been working through. I take the scalpel and make the opening in the baby's abdomen bigger. I put in the retractors and start looking around. I look at the stomach first, front and back. I can feel the inflated balloon at the end of the tube, right where it should be. There's no hole there. Maybe he's right. Maybe I'm just being paranoid. I follow the intestine from its junction with the stomach around the curve it makes where it attaches to the pancreas and the bile ducts.

"Flush the tube," I tell him, my eyes fixed to that spot. The water wells up, and at that instant I know exactly where it's coming from and how it got there. The tube must have been in too far when the balloon was inflated. Instead of being in the larger reservoir of the stomach, it was in the smaller diameter of the intestine. In the next instant the balloon was inflated, pulled back, and sutured into place. But at some point the fully expanded balloon ruptured the fragile thin-walled intestine. It's one of those complications I've only heard about before in one of Dr. R.'s medical disaster mini-lectures. And now it's my turn to come face-to-face with this complication, my technical error, my mistake, for the first time.

I reposition the retractors again and lift up the duodenum, the first part of the intestine. That's when I see the problem. From behind my magnifying glasses, it looks like a sinkhole that's opened up in the middle of a road, big enough to swallow an entire car. Although in reality it is only millimeters wide, I see only ragged edges and space where the smooth wall of the intestine used to be.

"Damn," I say, not quite believing what I am seeing. "How did this happen?"

I replay the sequence of events, who was holding what when the tube was inserted, how the tip got shoved in so far, how something like this happened. After the hundreds of feeding tubes I have done, each one executed in the exact same sequence, how did this happen, today, to this particular baby?

It is a question I will not be able to answer. Not today. Not ever. I will never know the exact moment the error took place, a fact that will unnerve me the next hundred times I do this procedure.

On February 12, 2009, Continental Connection Air Flight 3407 crashed near Buffalo, New York, killing all forty-nine people on board and one person on the ground. Neither pilot had slept in a bed the night before the flight. One pilot had slept in an airport lounge. Another pilot had taken an overnight cross-country flight riding in a jump seat before taking the helm as the plane's first officer.[4] Both pilots could be heard yawning on the plane's cockpit voice recorder. Pilot fatigue was cited as a major factor in the crash.

The families of the victims were outraged. There had been no major updates to pilot work schedule regulations since the 1960s, even though it was well documented that fatigue, like alcohol, can slow reflexes and impair judgment.[5] The National Transportation Safety Board had lobbied for two decades for new rules, but pilot unions and the airlines could not agree on what the limitations should be.

Finally, almost three years after the Buffalo crash, the Federal Aviation Administration (FAA) announced new rules that cap the maximum number of hours a pilot could be scheduled to fly to eight or nine (depending on the time of day and the time zones crossed) and mandated that passenger plane pilots sleep eight hours a day and take a minimum of ten hours off between shifts in the cockpit.[6]

Unfortunately, it had taken a tragedy to make the changes.

It is quite possible that exhaustion-related tragedies are happening every day in medicine, but we don't hear about them unless they are particularly egregious. While this is of heightened concern in skill-based specialties such as obstetrics and gynecology and surgery, other physicians are affected too, like those who are forced to respond to life-and-death situations in the emergency room and intensive care units.

Interns and residents (doctors in training) were the initial focus of advocates seeking to curtail work hours in the name of patient safety. A major catalyst in reforming resident work hours was the death of an eighteen-year-old woman in the New York Hospital in 1984.[7] Libby Zion was admitted with fever and extreme shaking that progressed to agitation. In the course of her treatment by junior residents who had been working all night, she was allegedly oversedated and died. Her father, a lawyer and newspaper columnist, filed a lawsuit, and not only publicized what happened to his daughter but also raised the profile of the public safety issues associated with being treated by overworked residents who worked thirty-six-hour shifts.[8]

For those of us who trained in the era of 100- to 120-hour workweeks, our on-call shifts would typically begin at 6 a.m. and end, if we were lucky, by 6 p.m. the following day — a total of thirty-six hours. We have vivid memories of feeling "punch drunk" by the time the next afternoon rolled around, fighting a heavy blanket of fatigue while struggling to stand upright in the operating room and hold on to retractors. We fell asleep at stoplights while driving home and nodded off at the dinner table or while talking on the phone. Sleep deprivation was the one characteristic that united all residents, no matter their specialty or year of training.

As Dr. Barron Lerner reflected twenty-five years after the fact, those of us in the trenches of residency training when the news of the Zion case hit were not surprised at the unfortunate mishap. We were just glad it hadn't happened to us.[9]

A study published in the *New England Journal of Medicine*, based on data collected before the work-hour reforms took place, found that error rates were 35 percent higher for interns who worked more frequent and longer shifts — in other words, a traditional schedule rather than a schedule that eliminated overnight shifts and reduced the total number of hours worked per week.[10]

Finally, in 2003, concerns over the rate of medical errors by sleep-deprived trainees ultimately forced the imposition of an eighty-hour workweek on residency training programs, including a thirty-hour limit on the length of any one shift. That meant that if a resident began work the prior day at 8 a.m., she would be off by noon the next day. A second wave of reforms (2009) mandated that interns were no longer allowed to work twenty-four-hour shifts.

Early studies tracking the medical error rate before and after the eighty-hour workweek went into effect have found that the number of medical errors did not fall.[11] While these results have been disappointing for proponents of the shorter workweek, several possible explanations have emerged. First, it is has been reported that up to two-thirds of residents regularly violate the eighty-hour restriction and work beyond their scheduled shifts. The second explanation is the patient handoff, a new wrinkle in patient care that resulted from work-hour restrictions. When residents were working longer shifts, there was more continuity of patient care. With shorter shifts come more frequent handoffs of responsibility for patient care from one resident to another. The more handoffs, the more potential for errors in communication regarding what tests must be ordered and checked on and other pressing issues in patient care.[12]

While the work hours of residents are restricted, there are no work-hour restrictions for attending physicians. Surgeons, for example, can work as many hours as they choose, from performing elective cases during the day to taking night call, even though studies show that exhausted surgeons, just like exhausted pilots, do not perform at their best. Medical error rates are higher for these surgeons than for those working fewer hours.[13]

In many call groups, one surgeon is routinely scheduled to work the entire weekend from Friday morning to Monday morning—a total of seventy-two hours. The surgeon would have absolutely no control over the volume of patients or phone calls she would be asked to handle during the weekend. She could work all day Friday performing a combination of elective and emergency cases. By Friday night, the surgeon could either still be in the hospital operating or at home in bed, where she would likely take phone calls from the nurses in the hospital, or from other doctors who need urgent consults, or from the emergency room about a patient who needs admission. Saturday would be spent performing more urgent and emergent operations and consulting on more patients. By the time Saturday evening rolled around, our weekend surgeon would be dragging, and might be groggy and confused when awakened, but her shift would continue for another thirty-six hours.

What are the results of such intense and pervasive sleep deprivation on performance? Studies have shown that an individual deprived of sleep for twenty-four hours has the same cognitive function as someone who is legally drunk.[14] The vigilance of three groups of subjects was compared over two weeks, with one group having eight hours of sleep a night, another group having six hours, and the third having four hours of sleep. While the eight-hour group had virtually no attention lapses, the reaction time of the six-hour and the four-hour groups declined steadily with each passing day, and by the end of the two weeks the six- and four-hour sleepers were as impaired as people who had been awake for twenty-four hours straight. What stands out is that even though fatigue was starting to affect performance, the subjects themselves perceived that sleepiness was not affecting them: in other words, people are poor judges of how much sleep they need.

Reducing nighttime sleep by as little as one and a half hours can decrease alertness by 32 percent.[15] Sleep deprivation predisposes individuals to numerous medical illnesses, including high blood pressure, heart attack, stroke, obesity, and psychiatric disorders.[16] During sleep the flow of cerebrospinal fluid around our brains increases dramatically and washes out toxic metabolites that build up when we are awake.[17] We all know the feeling of awaking refreshed after a good night's sleep compared with feeling sluggish and "off" when we've been up the night before. Yet despite the mounting evidence, surgeons continue to perform exacting operations in sleep-deprived states, when they are most vulnerable to making a mistake.

The assistant is deadly silent now as we assess the damage. He knows, like I do, that if we had closed the abdomen before finding this problem, we might well have killed the baby. Two things will make repairing the hole a challenge. First, we don't have much tissue to work with, and what we do have is tissue-paper thin. Just pulling the edges together enough to close the hole will be difficult. The second issue is that there are other very small tubular structures draining into the wall. We have to exercise the utmost care not to obstruct them as we close the hole. If we do, we will have an even bigger problem than the one we have now, one that could lead to lifelong complications or the patient's ultimate demise.

We start with the outer edges, carefully placing delicate, thin sutures in the wall and working our way toward the middle. When the hole is finally closed, I relax just a little, since the first, most difficult part is done. Then I fashion a patch over the repair with the omentum, the fatty apron of the abdomen; place a drain in case there is a leak; and close.

Like a quarterback who has just thrown a costly interception, I will not forgive myself until I know whether we have won or lost the game. I won't get any relief for a week or more, when I finally find out if everything has healed without yet another complication rising up to smack me in the face. In the meantime, my mistake will jog along beside me on the treadmill, where I blast it with the Rolling Stones. My mistake will sit next to me at dinner, where I will lose track of the conversation and stare out into space. My mistake will lull me to a fitful sleep and pepper my dreams.

When I wake up, I will repeatedly back the tape up to the point where no mistake has happened and make sure that none will happen again.

And I will think about Dr. R. and how he would weave this mistake into a lesson for trainees too naive to know the burdens of all the ways an operation can go wrong and how devastated a surgeon will feel when it does.

11

small

Imagine being asked to operate on a patient you cannot examine, a patient floating in a small, dark, murky container. You will be working underwater. You will not be able to keep him entirely still, move him into optimal position before cutting, or attach to his body any of the standard monitoring devices, such as EKG leads.

Now imagine that this patient is one-hundredth the size of the average human, no bigger than a day-old Labrador puppy, six inches long and weighing about a pound. You'll be attempting this risky procedure, which may end your patient's life, at just over the halfway mark in gestation. His organs—heart, liver, kidneys—will be smaller than Lego bricks and infinitely more delicate. Oh, and this patient you're about to attempt this procedure on, he's inside another human being, his mother. You'll have to cut through her first to get to him and then find your way into her uterus, which, by the way, does not like to be messed with. The finicky organ might punish the entire endeavor by launching into a reckless paroxysm of contractions that kicks your patient out early, as in tomorrow, which will be more than enough to do him in, because he will be far too premature to survive.

These are the baseline conditions that challenge fetal surgeons in every undertaking, operating on the slim edge that separates the feasible from the unthinkable. They must traverse three unique physiologic environments—the mother's body, the womb, and, finally, the developing human—just to get to the body part that needs to be repaired, and they must do so with a degree of precision that allows no room for error.

What makes this possible?

Fetal surgery in the 1970s was science fiction, an imagined therapy dependent on scientific advances yet to be made that existed somewhere in the future and in the mind of Dr. Michael Harrison, a young surgeon training in Boston. To him the concept made perfect sense. The newborn congenital anomalies that pediatric surgeons operated on were almost always the result of developmental errors that occurred during pregnancy. If an abnormality could be detected and repaired early enough to prevent the downstream, often fatal, consequences, perhaps a future could be altered and a baby's life saved.

Fetal intervention was not entirely unheard-of at the time. In the early 1960s, Sir William Liley, a New Zealand perinatologist, had successfully transfused a fetus to treat hydrops fetalis, a frequently fatal condition induced by Rh blood group incompatibility between the mother and fetus.[1] This amazing feat, which predated the widespread availability of prenatal ultrasound, was carried out using X-rays and contrast infusion to guide the accurate placement of a needle into the abdominal cavity of the fetus.[2] Around this same time there were reported attempts in New York and Puerto Rico to directly access the fetal circulation by opening the womb to access the jugular and femoral veins of a fetus. Due to the disappointing results, however, operating on the fetus was abandoned and would not be resurrected for over a decade.[3]

Pediatric surgery had been stretching the boundaries of operative candidates to include younger and smaller patients. Even extremely premature infants, whose features were more fetal-like than full-scale human, could tolerate operations surprisingly well if a surgeon was careful and didn't try to do too much. Fetal surgery was, in a way, the logical next step, albeit one that posed unique hazards to both mother and fetus, generating concerns that would vex medical ethicists and provide a treasure trove of material to comment on for decades to come.

The main ethical dilemma swirled around the fact that the mother was an innocent bystander in any therapy attempted on the fetus. There was no direct benefit for the mother, but if the fetus was going under the knife, she would have to also. The risks of general anesthesia and bleeding from the uterus and placenta, both highly vascular organs, were significant and could be life-threatening to both participants. The mother would also have to undergo two cesarean sections: one for the fetal intervention and another one later to deliver the baby as close to term as possible. To some, putting the mother at risk was simply not acceptable, especially for what might turn out to be a nonviable pregnancy.

If a surgeon was looking for a challenge, a hostile environment in which to practice his craft, fetal surgery was a good place to start. The gravid uterus was a hungry pit bull on steroids—unpredictable and looking for a fight. Simply cutting and inserting instruments into the uterine wall was enough to cause contractions and initiate early labor and premature delivery. Uterine contractions would have to be muzzled if fetal surgery was ever going to succeed.

Another roadblock was the placenta, an engorged tangle of blood vessels attached to the inside of the uterus. Even a tiny nick could cause a flood of uncontrollable hemorrhage, interrupt the fetus's lifeline, and cause certain death. Like the restricted airspace of an enemy country, surgeons would need to map the placental borders and steer completely around them to avoid potential catastrophe.

The fetus, like any surgical patient, would require monitoring during the operation. Surgeons would need to know if the fetal heart rate was slowing, the oxygen level was low, and the fetus was moving. The fetus was connected to its own life support—the maternal circulation—but that was no guarantee of safety.

The fetus remained vulnerable to placental malfunctions, premature delivery, or sudden death from other causes. New techniques to monitor a patient that could not be easily touched would have to be developed.

Nothing defined the field of fetal surgery so much as danger, risk, and controversy. It was no surprise, therefore, that an avalanche of skepticism greeted Harrison's proposal that fetal surgery might be feasible, but he was not easily thrown off the scent. He eventually made his way west to San Francisco, where he found open and innovative minds to share in his vision.[4] He formed a specialized team of fetal experts at the University of California at San Francisco, which included maternal-fetal specialists, obstetrical radiologists, anesthesiologists, and neonatologists.

Harrison would still need to lay the groundwork for the field, painstakingly reproducing human anomalies in animals and then devising operations that could be performed with a minimum of disruption to a human-in-progress. Up to that point, what little was known about this tiniest of patients, the fetus, had mostly been discovered through observation and mishaps. There was still a lot to learn about the fetal anatomy, organ function in utero compared to that in full-term newborns, and how much a fetus could tolerate in the way of intervention. There was no handbook for this sort of thing. Harrison and his coworkers would have to literally discover almost every aspect of what it took to operate on a fetus and write the book on their own.[5]

But along the way they would encounter critics, naysayers lurking in the wings and anxious to shut down the production before the curtain had even begun to rise.

"The mood now of the physicians is it should not be done," a prominent physician from Boston commented. "It should not be done thinking it's therapy."[6]

The prevailing attitude among Harrison's team, therefore, was that if fetal surgery was going to be done, it must be done the right way to avoid the perception of being daring and reckless—

to always put the mother's health first, methodically investigate methods in the laboratory before applying them to living breathing humans, and take every precaution to minimize risk to both mother and unborn baby.

Given the inherent risk of intervention, Harrison's team confined their initial work to treating only life-threatening conditions. They started with relatively simple anatomic defects that had devastating consequences to the developing fetus, such as congenital diaphragmatic hernia, a hole in the diaphragm that kept the lungs from developing properly; urinary tract obstructions that could stifle kidney and lung development; and spina bifida, a gap in the covering of the spine that caused paralysis.

The fetal period extends from the ninth week of gestation to birth. During this time most of the fetal tissues are maturing so organs can function when a baby is born. The body is also growing rapidly during this time. The face develops more human characteristics during the twelfth week. During the sixteenth to twentieth weeks, still the first half of gestation, the fetus lengthens rapidly. During the second half of gestation, from the twentieth week on, the fetus gains weight.

In order to change the outcome of the developing fetus by the time of birth, most operations need to be undertaken at twenty-two to twenty-five weeks of gestation, when the fetus is about half the size of a full-term infant. At this early stage the skin is wrinkled and emits a reddish glow from the network of capillaries surging just beneath the tissue-thin surface. Subcutaneous fat has not yet been deposited. The eyes are still fused. If a baby is born at six months, approximately twenty-four weeks of gestation, it will have a difficult time surviving because the organ systems are not yet able to fully function.[7] The fetal surgeon must work in this window between inability to survive and viability, understanding that the fetus is inherently the smallest and most physiologically vulnerable patient a pediatric surgeon will ever have, and no matter what precautions are taken, every procedure is extremely high risk.

Harrison's first successful clinical intervention came in 1981. The mother was seven months pregnant, carrying twins. Only one twin's life was in danger, however.

The male fetus had posterior urethral valves, a condition in which the passage of urine from the bladder into the amnion is blocked. His abdomen was swelling so much from the retained fluid that the pressure on the diaphragms kept his lungs from developing. The back pressure on his kidneys would cause renal dysplasia, a stifling of the growth and function of the kidneys, by the time he was born. Still, the risk/benefit ratio was high, as the procedure was experimental and the outcome difficult to predict. What clouded the picture even more was that doctors feared that performing a procedure on the male fetus might put the female fetus's life at risk too.

"The twin sister posed an ethical dilemma," Harrison later recalled. "We were just in agony at the time."[8]

At twenty-eight weeks of gestation, Harrison inserted a custom-made catheter into the obstructed bladder of the male fetus.[9] The shunt worked, draining urine into the amniotic fluid and decompressing the bladder. The child survived the procedure and went on to live a normal life. A quarter of a century later the two met again in Harrison's office. His patient was now a young college student and displayed few ill effects from the in utero abnormality that had once threatened his future.

Not every attempt at repair would be successful in those early days. Some promising procedures were shelved or abandoned when they did not prove worth the risk compared to conventional postnatal therapy.[10] One major disappointment was a clinical trial that was undertaken in the mid-1980s to investigate the in utero repair of diaphragmatic hernia. The trial ultimately demonstrated that in utero intervention was no better than conventional treatment after birth.

This setback, however, steered Harrison's group toward developing a new approach. Instead of concentrating on the anatomic defect and patching the hole in the diaphragm, Harrison attacked what was killing the baby: the fact that the lungs were underdeveloped because they were being compressed by intestine that had slid into the chest. Inserting a plug into the trachea of fetal lambs generated airway pressure that would force the lungs to grow.

While the laboratory results were promising, the treatment again failed to improve the survival of infants with the condition under the rigors of a randomized trial reported in 2002. But what looked like a defeat from the outside turned out to be just a starting point. Modifications of the tracheal plug procedure led to more promising outcomes in Europe. With the more refined technique and the benefit of ten more years of clinical experience, it is likely the procedure will ultimately prove to offer a significant benefit.

Harrison's group went on to develop techniques to treat other conditions in the fetus—abdominal tumors, twin-twin vascular anomalies, lung malformations, and neck masses. They were one of the first to use fetoscopy, the use of a tiny fiber-optic telescope that measures 1–2 millimeters (3/100th of an inch) through which the fetus can be viewed. Fetoscopy allows the placement of equally tiny instruments through bendable straw-sized tubes inserted into micro-incisions. Fetal surgery performed through these small tubes is a major improvement over procedures performed through a large opening in the uterus that could induce preterm labor. Some procedures, in fact, were so well tolerated that they could be performed under local anesthesia and the mother discharged the same day.

Harrison made fetal surgery a reality. Along the way he brought young, inquisitive surgeons into his lab for years at a time and eventually dispersed his disciples like spores out into the world to populate future fetal surgery centers. More amazing feats would be accomplished by his protégés that would touch the lives of countless infants. This lineage started with a vision inside one man's head, a man with the personal fortitude to withstand the critique of mainstream surgery. When the bulk of the tedious work had been done and the barriers to entering the fetal surgery business had been lowered, surgeons across the country would try to emulate Harrison's model of a fetal treatment center.

The impetus for fetal surgery was inextricably tied to the development of prenatal ultrasound—a safe, noninvasive test that allowed obstetricians to diagnose in utero anatomic abnormalities and prompted surgeons to contemplate repairing them.

The first ultrasound machines grew out of a serendipitous encounter between an obstetrician and a businessman. In 1954, Dr. Ian Donald, an obstetrician and gynecologist in Glasgow, performed a hysterectomy on a patient whose husband had ties to a company that manufactured boilers for the shipbuilding industry.[11] The boilermakers used an industrial flaw detector, a primitive form of ultrasound, to look for cracks beneath the surface of a boiler.

After seeing the instrument for the first time, Donald reportedly returned to the factory with a trunk full of pathology specimens—a uterus with fibroids, an ovary with a large cyst, and various other body parts—to investigate using the machine. For the first time he could discern pathology beneath the surface of an organ without cutting into it.

The first ultrasound machines (the A-type) were similar to underwater radar detectors or sonar that would display a blip on an oscilloscope screen when an object was detected. Ultrasound images are produced by bouncing high-frequency sound waves off the surface of an object and visualizing the echoes or waves reflected back by internal structures. As soon as Donald could get his hands on an A-type machine, he started using ultrasound in his practice to examine patients with suspected abdominal and pelvic masses.

Tom Brown, an engineer with an interest in ultrasound, joined Donald and was later credited with developing the next generation of ultrasound machines, the two-dimensional ultrasound. In 1957, the first known ultrasound studies of a human fetus took place when Donald and Brown discovered a fetus by accident in a patient with an enlarged uterus.[12]

In the early 1960s prenatal ultrasound was available in only a few major medical centers, including the University of Colorado, where Dr. Joseph Holmes, known as the "father of ultrasound," was developing his own machine and making major contributions to the field. He was joined by Dr. Horace Thompson, who focused on the diagnostic applications in obstetrics. Ultrasound machines were also being tested in Sweden, Japan, Austria, and a handful of other centers in the United States.[13]

In 1965, an international symposium on diagnostic ultrasound was held in Pittsburgh, where numerous papers on the obstetrical applications of ultrasound were presented. This marked the turning point for the acceptance of ultrasound as a proven technique with unique clinical applications. The next year Blue Cross/Blue Shield authorized reimbursement for medical ultrasound, and other insurance companies quickly followed its lead. By the mid- to late 1960s, ultrasound was becoming widely available throughout the United States and around the world.

Ultrasound was an ideal tool to examine the fetus, as it was noninvasive and posed no known risk and, unlike X-rays, did not subject the fetus to ionizing radiation. Before the advent of fetal surgery, ultrasound had been used to guide needle placement into umbilical cord vessels to perform in utero transfusions. With ultrasound guidance, needles could be inserted into the uterus to sample the amniotic fluid (amniocentesis) and to obtain biopsies of skin and liver from the fetus for diagnostic purposes.[14]

Imaging techniques such as two- and three-dimensional ultrasound and real-time, in-the-moment imaging have become more refined over the past few decades. Ultrasound has evolved from a crude imaging technique turning out grainy black-and-white images in which the outlines of the fetal silhouette could barely be recognized, to a technique that can discern the anatomy of a fetal mouse heart at nine days of gestation—structures as small as 30 microns, roughly equivalent to a grain of pollen.[15]

Fetal magnetic resonance scanning (MRI), introduced in the 1990s, provides even greater resolution than ultrasound. It is particularly useful for delineating the anatomy of the developing brain and spinal cord. One drawback initially was that to obtain a detailed anatomic rendering the patient had to be completely still, a condition that can be difficult to achieve with a fetus. But newer, so-called "fast" MRI techniques, produce high-quality images even in the face of movement.

Fetal interventionists currently utilize ultrasound to guide the insertion of needles, fetoscopes, and percutaneous instruments during closed procedures. Real-time three-dimensional imaging via ultrasound and MRI provide even greater anatomical detail to guide surgeons in planning and executing complicated procedures.

Very few people have heard of congenital anomalies until they're seeing a specialist because of an abnormal prenatal ultrasound. I meet the parents in my office before the starting gun of birth has even sounded—an earnest couple, holding hands, listening to every word. On the day the mother had a routine prenatal ultrasound fifteen weeks into pregnancy, the only new information they were hoping to leave with was the sex of the baby and the usual reassuring "ten fingers, ten toes."

When the test was finished, however, they were asked to go back to the waiting room because there was something the obstetrician might want to discuss with them. That was the day things started to go wrong, the day they found out that their baby's blueprint had gone awry. Now these two unfortunate parents were lost in the dense woods of medical jargon and YouTube videos, left to obsessively scan the Internet for hopeful news and a hint of what was to come. They never expected this when they decided to

start a family, and now they were looking to me to lead them out
. . . if there was a path.

*Yes, there is a problem. We can see it right here on the ultrasound
just like the technician showed you in that dark room where your belly
was slick with lubricant while she pushed in and rubbed the white
plastic wand from side to side.*

Most of the time when a patient comes in for a prenatal consul-
ation the defect can be repaired, but when a baby was missing the
entire left side of his diaphragm or had a massive tumor that was
robbing the fetal circulation and damaging other organs, or in the
rare event it was something I had never seen before and had no
idea how to treat, I was going to have to edit that speech. I studied the grainy ultrasound snapshots, read the obstetrician's notes,
and looked at everything two or three times, because I wanted to
be sure before the words left my mouth.

"This could be rougher than the usual case," I said, "but I can
promise you we will try everything that modern medicine has to
offer."

That was the point where truth met up with reality, because
modern medicine didn't have a cure for everyone. There would always be those we could not fix, the ones we got to too late, months
after the dominos had tumbled into the chaos of a devastating and
irreversible malformation. We would open the baby up and puzzle out the anatomy, and then it would hit us. The cards the baby
had been dealt, the cards left for us to play, were a losing hand.
We were not going to leave the operating room puffed up and tri-
umphant today.

There was no way to fix the abnormality and no way to bring
this painful episode to a close. The situation would have to play
out when the baby was born, the disappointment weighing on the
family like a tow chain dragging them mercilessly through days,
weeks, or longer as the grief that accompanies all bad outcomes
swelled and broke through the surface of their denial.

Surgeons were bred to weather the most brutal of scenarios without so much as a grimace. But would I sleep that night? Would I be able to stop the constant loop replay of every move I had and hadn't made? Would I ever forget this baby, his mother and father, his extinguished what-might-have-been?

I first encountered the congenital spine abnormality spina bifida as an intern assisting a pediatric neurosurgeon in repairing myelo-meningoceles, the most common type. Spina bifida, a hole in the spine, is a defect that occurs during the first month of pregnancy, in many cases before a woman even knows she's pregnant. The baby may look perfectly normal from the front, but when you turn him over there is a translucent nerve-filled sac protruding from the lower back, like a small jellyfish, not particularly menacing in appearance but with devastating consequences for a child — lower extremity paralysis, intestinal and bladder dysfunction, a loss of sensation and a permanent loss of nerve function from the level of the defect to everything below it. Because the brain and the spinal cord are connected and the brain too may have abnor-malities, the most severely affected babies usually developed hy-drocephalus and required a tube in the brain to drain the fluid.

The only operation available in the 1990s was to close the dura, the outer lining around the spinal cord, and cover the gap by stretching nearby muscle and skin and closing these layers over for extra strength. Closing the hole was easy, but it would not re-store the nerves that had been damaged in utero, while the spi-nal cord and nerves were bathed in amniotic fluid and became scarred and snarled.

Spina bifida wasn't necessarily a life-threatening diagnosis, but it was a life-altering one for which there was no cure. There was no way to restore a spinal cord once it had been scarred by the in utero exposure to amniotic fluid. The nerve damage was permanent.

Later in my pediatric surgery fellowship I rotated through the spina bifida clinic. Children of all ages were brought in, some in wheelchairs, some on stretchers, some on crutches, very few able to ambulate without some kind of assistance. The clinic hallway reeked of urine and stool because they were all incontinent. Their charts were thick as an LA phonebook, and their X-ray jackets were splitting at the seams.

It would take a platoon of physicians to sort out all the medical and surgical issues — pediatricians who specialized in chronic disease, neurosurgeons who operated on the brain and spine, neurologists who tracked neurologic impairment, urologists who dealt with bladders that could not empty, orthopedic surgeons who could address lower limb deformities, and pediatric surgeons who could troubleshoot gastrostomy tubes and central lines. The one thing all the patients had in common was that they would be living with this condition for the rest of their lives, many of which would be cut short by the complications of hydrocephalus, kidney impairment, or a sudden, overwhelming infection. Other than administering lifelong supportive care, there was no way to change their fate.

Spina bifida tempted fetal surgeons to revise their criteria for intervention because it was a relatively simple anatomic defect — a hole — that might be amenable to a very simple fix. Yes, technically this anomaly wasn't life-threatening, but it was a devastating defect that could not be cured. Before fetal surgery to repair the defect could be added to the acceptable reasons to operate in utero, a question had to be answered. If surgeons got to the defect early enough and patched it like a blown-out tire, would this prevent the extensive nerve damage usually seen after birth?

To answer the question a research study would have to be undertaken, a controlled clinical trial where patients voluntarily enrolled and were randomly placed into one group that got the fetal operation and another group that didn't. The outcomes of the two groups would then be compared. Conducting such a study would not be easy. Half of those carrying a child with the defect who enrolled in the study would be giving up a shot at the only known prenatal treatment. Because only a select few fetal surgery centers could participate in the trial, some centers currently performing the procedure would have to agree to a moratorium until the trial was concluded and the results known.

The NIH-funded, $22.5 million study was started in 2003 and continued until the results were pointing unfailingly in one direction.[16] At this point 160 patients had been enrolled: 80 were selected for surgery after birth, and 80 had the spinal opening closed in utero. As it turned out, those who had the prenatal procedure were half as likely to have brain complications and had much better motor function in their legs. Many would be able to walk even without crutches. The results were so dramatic that the study was stopped—but this time it was because of success, not failure. It would be ethically wrong to continue to assign the patients blindly to one group or the other. Every fetus diagnosed with spina bifida should be considered for fetal intervention if they met the criteria and their parents consented.

Fetal surgery resembles the space program in at least two regards. Like the space program, where some missions were considered a success and others frank disasters, fetal surgery has had its share of victories and defeats and even now has perhaps not fulfilled all of its promise. But as with the space program, the technological spin-offs from years of bright young minds studying the fetus and trying to perfect the procedures have been impressive in their own right.

One such spin-off was the EXIT procedure, a specialized delivery technique employed when babies were diagnosed prenatally with airway compression from a congenital anomaly such as a mouth or neck tumor.[17] This procedure was originally developed to reverse the temporary tracheal occlusion that Harrison's group used to treat severe cases of in utero diaphragmatic hernia.

An EXIT procedure is performed during a cesarean section. The baby is scooped up out of the uterus and placed on the operating table next to the mother still attached to the placenta, which acts as a heart-lung bypass machine while the airway of the baby is examined and a tube placed to secure ventilation. While the technique of tracheal occlusion is still being investigated in clinical trials, the EXIT has been applied to a wide variety of conditions during which a baby might suffer respiratory distress from airway obstruction.

Fetoscopy allows manipulation of the fetus without opening the uterus.[18] Another particularly useful spin-off has been the development of tiny fetoscopes, some measuring as small as 1.5 millimeters, roughly the width of a matchstick, that can be inserted into the uterus to visualize abnormalities and assist in their repair. The availability of fetoscopy allows fetal surgery to be performed without opening the uterus, thereby lowering the incidence of complications such as bleeding and preterm labor.

More advances have been made in controlling preterm labor, monitoring the fetus remotely during procedures, and limiting bleeding while opening the uterus. All of these advances have broader applications to obstetrics beyond fetal surgery and have helped improve the care of all pregnant patients.

Thirty years into fetal surgery, much progress has been made, but still there are only an estimated five hundred procedures performed per year in the United States.[19] While there are only a handful of major fetal surgery centers—San Francisco, Philadelphia, and Vanderbilt—programs are springing up across the country, and at last count there were at least fifteen hospitals offering fetal surgery.

Despite the refinement in tools and techniques, and in some cases because of them, controversies abound in fetal surgery. How many fetal surgery centers should there be in our country? Congenital anomalies are rare to begin with, and those with operative indications represent a mere sliver. It takes a certain number

of cases to gain and maintain the technical proficiency necessary to have satisfactory treatment results. Does it make sense
to dilute the existing pool of patients across numerous centers?
What are the minimal numbers of cases that a fetal surgery center needs to have sufficient expertise, and who will monitor and
accredit them?

What are the minimal resources that a fetal surgery center
should have on hand? For example, how many fetal surgeons,
maternal-fetal obstetricians, and specially trained nurses and as-
sistants are required to perform these operations and monitor the
patients afterward? What type of specialized equipment, including that required for specialized fetal imaging, will be required?
What type of institutions can and will make the investment necessary to maintain the programs with the highest-quality outcomes?

A recent report reviewing the state of available published research on the outcomes of fetal surgery concluded that the ability
to perform fetal operations has "gotten ahead of the research."[20]
The report raised concerns about the active marketing of fetal
procedures that offered hope for a successful outcome when the
published results were still inconclusive.

Many fetal surgery operations have not yet been proven to
be effective by clinical trials. Should these be undertaken at all?
Should they be decided on a case-by-case basis? Should every proposed procedure undergo the rigors and delay of a prospective
randomized trial? For the most unusual defects there may not
be adequate numbers to justify or support a clinical trial. Does it
make sense to deny patients the benefit of these procedures if, in
the judgment of surgeon, there is a chance of success?

As the technology and indications for fetal intervention expand, the question remains who decides which patients should
have the procedures and who will pay for them. Insurance companies typically do not pay for experimental procedures, and
fetal specialists have battled with them over the years. For some

conditions, such as diaphragmatic hernia, that are still as yet un-proven, there may be some potential cost savings to be gained in an early intervention that prevents weeks to months in a neona-tal intensive care unit. For other conditions the cost benefits are not so clear, and the results are no more certain than a coin flip.

Progress has been made in identifying in utero abnormalities ear-lier in gestation and devising interventions with the benefit of better imaging, anesthesia, and tools. What is not always clear, however, is whether the benefits of most procedures outweigh the risks of prenatal intervention. Harrison himself published a fetal surgery report card in 2002 in which the success of most proce-dures was graded as average and many were deemed failures or near failures.

"It is now clear that because a procedure can be done does not mean it should be done and that a fetal abnormality of any type should never be treated simply 'because it is there,'" Harrison stated, summing up the state of fetal surgery.[21]

Following Harrison's lead, his disciples continue to insist on scientific rigor in deciding when and if certain procedures should be performed. A guiding principle has been that when a better way emerges, one that does not require invasive surgery and is less risky to the fetus, it should be welcomed. There should be no turf battle when it comes to the safety of the mother and child.

Fetal surgery has emerged as a recognized specialty, with a pro-fessional society of specialists, a journal, and a textbook. The in-dications for fetal intervention are projected to further expand in scope and locations across the country. Harrison has stressed, however, that fetal surgeons need to be honest with prospective parents, as there are still many uncertainties associated with the procedures, their outcomes, and the overall risk.

With all the attendant trials and tribulations a new reality has emerged from the fetal surgery era: the fetus is no longer hidden away in her mother's uterus beyond the reach of medical care. No matter how small, this most vulnerable of humans is a potential patient, one who has captured the imagination of surgeons dedicated to rerouting gestational detours so a child can have a shot at a normal life.

12

the lost and found

At three in the morning on Christmas Eve we meet for the first time, sitting side by side in bolted-to-the-floor faded turquoise chairs. You are the father of a newborn who needs an emergency operation, as in *right now*. Your baby, just three days old, is being wheeled through the halls of the hospital en route to an operating room one floor below, where he will be put to sleep and readied for an exploration of his abdomen.

I am your baby's surgeon, someone who should be dashing down the hall after his isolette, but first I must talk to you, and it is not going to be easy. These attempts to explain sudden catastrophe and what comes next are never easy. In residency we referred to chats like this as "hanging crepe," as in black crepe draped across the steam engine of Lincoln's funeral train. If you have managed to cling to any shred of denial up to this point, I'm about to peel it away like a burn victim's scorched skin from the underlying flesh, leaving the nerve endings raw and exposed. Christmas, scalpels, dead gut — a cruel and awkward combination of realities at best, a disaster at worst.

Fate has pressed us together on these hard plastic chairs, under the unflinching gaze of fluorescent lights, looking down at the stained linoleum floor. Me, an overworked surgeon emerging from a deep sleep, stoked by adrenaline surging through my veins, and you, a person who could be my brother-in-law, the captain of the football team, the neighbor two houses down who mows his yard on the weekends. Your eyes, puffy and red, lock onto mine.

Oh, God, not this guy tonight, I think. *Not a guy sitting here in his Dockers, polo shirt, and sockless loafers whom I can relate to without even trying. How will I ever stand to tell him if this doesn't turn out well?*

I have the unfortunate but necessary obligation to tell you that your firstborn, your son, your Christmas baby, anticipated with all the hope and joy one person can hold for another, may not make it out of the operating room alive. I hate to even think the words, much less speak them, after everything you've been through. You deserve respite, reassurance, relief—but I can't offer any, only a sliver of hope and not much more. Just like you have no choice about what you're going to hear in the next ten minutes, I have no choice about what I'm going to say.

Riding my own roller coaster through long stretches that leave me crumpled and drained, I know about stress, disappointment, and defeat: but even on my worst days I will in no way be facing the hell you are this holiday season. First your baby, misidentified as "healthy" at delivery, was relabeled within hours as "extremely unstable," with a probable heart defect. The defect was not anything as simple as a hole between the chambers that might close on its own. It was something much worse: truncus arteriosus, a rare condition in which the main arteries feeding the lungs and the body fail to separate during gestation. It is a serious heart malformation, one that can be repaired with a major operation but that has moved to the back burner at the moment. He has to make it through this more imminent threat first.

The bad news just keeps coming, rumbling along, funneling us like traffic past an accident scene to this rushed and regrettable introduction. You'll spend more time with the clerk who checks your groceries or the teller at the drive-through window than you will with me, a complete stranger, before I cut your baby open and preside over what could be the ultimate event in his life.

I know the scenes that have been flashing before your eyes like some kind of big-screen action adventure movie you'd rather not have a part in — the helicopter transfer to a children's hospital in a strange city, the urgent echocardiogram, the heart defect diagnosis, and, as if that wasn't enough, now this unexpected surprise. A few hours after arriving here, your son started vomiting, his belly swelling to ripe-melon firmness. His skin blanched a deathly pale. His blood pressure began to dive as he gasped for breath. He looked like he was trying to die.

The NICU team jumped on him, swarming his bed, poking a million times to get another IV, inserting a breathing tube. A loud boxy machine that looked like a prop from a Cold War–era documentary, rolled up to the bed for X-rays. Five minutes later those films were developed and showed the classic bubbling in the wall of the intestine that pointed to a severe case of necrotizing enterocolitis, a disease that destroys the intestine of vulnerable newborns. Worse still, there was a pocket of air outside the intestinal wall indicating that some portion had already died and started leaking toxic bacteria into your son's no-longer-sterile abdomen.

That was when I was called and the two of us were put on a path that led to the place we are now, sitting on these two uncomfortable low-bid relics, as unyielding as the situation we find ourselves in. I give a condensed version of the usual speech I deliver when I'm about to operate on a baby who is crashing like a 737 with hydraulics failure and only one possible ending, unwritten but virtually certain. I leave you in stunned silence and promise to return.

Thirty minutes later I am staring at the answer. As the tip of the knife dives below the peritoneal lining, brown fluid, always a terrible sign, spouts out and splashes my gloved hand. The unmistakable putrid stench of dead gut mixed with anaerobic bacteria wafts up through the turbid swirl. The intestine is pale yellow splotched with purple, the dead patches already liquefying in my hands. I extend the incision to the right, then to the left, finding only more of the same dead and dying scraps, blown out through and through, floating in a stew of stool and blood.

The worst possible feeling washes over me — *I am not going to be able to save this baby.* The impending dread of the next impossible task quickly follows — going out to those chairs again to find the boy next door and tell him.

Even with the words silently rehearsed I cannot stop the grief that wells up every single time I have to tell a parent that a child is on the verge of dying. This loss that will shape and haunt the parents' lives forever will remain a part of mine also. This death will land in the same place where the others are recorded, ready to unfurl like a banner every time another name joins the list.

I go out to the hallway to find my patient's father. His face is a question suffused with a hope that mine cannot return.

"The news is not good," I tell him. "We could only open and close."

He hangs his head in his outstretched hands and weeps.

Surgeons live with the conundrum of lost body parts because they, by definition, are the ones who take them out. Some organs are lost to a disease like cancer, others to injury, unfortunate events that can happen almost anytime during the seventy-five-year life expectancy of the average American. Of all the surgeons removing organs, however, pediatric surgeons are most often confronted with the added complexity of working on patients who are missing organs early in life.

Standing in the operating room at the moment of discovery, questions reel through a pediatric surgeon's mind like breaking news scrolling across the bottom of a CNN broadcast. *Can the child survive without this missing part? What can I use in its place? What can I do to temporize the situation until a more permanent solution becomes available? Will this solution/patch/repair grow with the baby, or will it have to be replaced in a year or two?*

The pediatric surgeon can't simply take inventory and close. She has to figure out a substitute for what's missing, and that usually means finding a way to reconstruct/borrow/improvise an organ or tissue structure, with the goal of providing the child with as close to a normal life as possible.

Even now, in an era when we routinely replace joints and heart valves, install pacemakers and defibrillators and have even invented a prosthetic limb that will allow an amputee to compete in the Olympics, there is still no artificial substitute for the small intestine.

In Robert Gross's 1953 textbook, *The Surgery of Infancy and Childhood*, there is a photograph of a group of hospitalized children ranging in age from newborns to toddlers. All of these children had something in common. They were born without something they needed to be able to eat — an intact esophagus. The caption reads: *Photograph of 9 children who were simultaneously in the hospital for treatment of esophageal atresia.*[1] Esophageal atresia, a condition where the swallowing tube was blocked at birth and might have an abnormal connection to the trachea, was one of the first reconstructive challenges pediatric surgeons attempted.

In the 1940s, it was understood that many infants would not leave the hospital with a functioning esophagus after the initial diagnosis of esophageal atresia. A child could survive without an esophagus but would need to be fed directly into the stomach through a tube, and could not eat by mouth until the two ends of the esophagus were joined. Depending on their overall condition children might stay in the hospital for months to years undergoing a series of operations to reconstruct the esophagus. As Gross himself wrote, there were "enormous technical difficulties, requiring infinite patience on the part of the surgeon and the patient."[2] The lengths of hospitalization would extend for months or even several years.

The predominant technique used to repair esophageal atresia

was known as "antethoracic esophageal reconstruction," because the esophagus would be rebuilt outside the chest cavity, just under the skin overlying the chest wall.[3] The upper esophagus was frequently constructed with a tube of skin and subcutaneous tissue, causing an unsightly bulge in the upper chest. The lower esophagus was constructed from a piece of small intestine that was isolated and sewn to the stomach on the lower end and to the skin tube at the upper end. A tube made out of skin, however, could not propel food through like a native esophagus, and children would occasionally have to use their hands to massage the tube to move a bolus of swallowed food down to their stomachs. This procedure was never attempted on a newborn. The reconstruction was put off for months or years, until the child was larger, with the assumption that the operation and anesthesia would be better tolerated in an older child.

By the 1950s, newer techniques were developed that allowed the two ends of the esophagus to be joined within the chest. Today a baby with esophageal atresia might have a repair shortly after birth and go home within a week, thanks to advances in anesthesia, antibiotics, neonatal intensive care, and innovative surgical techniques. Ingenious operations have been devised to solve the problem of an esophagus that won't reach. If the two ends of the esophagus were too short to join together, the most logical substitute was some other part of the gastrointestinal tract. The intestine was the tissue most like the esophagus, with a smooth lining known as the mucosa and an outer muscular layer that could, theoretically, move the swallowed food through the chest and into the stomach.

Small intestine, colon, and stomach have been used as substitutes, but no matter what material or technique is used, nothing functions as well as the one complete esophagus babies should be born with, and there is still a group of affected children who cannot undergo successful primary repair. There will be some complicating factor such as other medical problems or anomalies, or ends of the esophagus that are so far apart they cannot be re-connected.

I first met Mitzi when she was six months old, sitting up, watching multicolored Teletubbies dancing on the TV screen above her bed. The intermittent hiss of the ventilator that breathed for her filled the room. A constant stream of drool dripped from the corner of her mouth. A tube whitened by milky formula snaked into her stomach for feedings.

Still, she was clapping and smiling. This was the only life she'd ever known. This bed, these four walls, the doctors, nurses, and respiratory therapists who came and went at the change of shift were her de facto family, replacing the parents who had never returned. She didn't know it should have been easier, that she could have been born some other way and been at home with an attentive mother, sitting in her own high chair, dumping strained peas on the floor with every other bite.

Instead, the inside of Mitzi's chest was so jumbled when she was born it was like the instruction manual had been misplaced when it was her turn to be put together. Her esophagus ended somewhere just past her neck, way short of the stomach, where it should have connected. Her heart had holes between the major chambers. The blood heading back to her lungs traveled through small threadlike arteries rather than the wide-open conduits most people had.

Mitzi's first operation was performed on her second day of life to separate her esophagus from her trachea, an abnormal connection that let spit and gastric contents seep into her lungs and cause low-grade pneumonia. After opening, the surgeon located the short end of the esophagus, a brownish finger-sized pouch lodged high in the chest. He pulled it gently with his forceps and worked it away from the surrounding tissue, but it couldn't be coaxed to join to the matching nub on the stomach. It was too short, and no amount of maneuvering would bring it down.

Mitzi was far too small and had other life-threatening problems, like her heart, that could act up and drop her oxygen levels in a hurry. Weighing barely four pounds, she could not withstand a major reconstruction. All the surgeon could do was mark the two ends and close. The esophageal reconnection would have to wait until another day, with the hope that the two ends would grow over the ensuing months and that with time they could be connected. In the meantime, Mitzi sat with a large plastic tube down her throat to suck out the saliva that otherwise drooled out the corner of her mouth. Without a passage to the stomach, eating was out of the question. She would have to be fed through a gastrostomy tube that inserted directly into her stomach.

A few weeks after the first operation, she had another one, this time on her heart to bypass the twiglike arteries to her lungs. The procedure was just a temporary solution, but it was the only option for a baby with a heart the size of a snapper turtle's, not yet big enough to undergo an operation that would definitively correct the problem.

With a marginally repaired heart and chronic lung disease from aspirating saliva, Mitzi became dependent on the ventilator. Her third operation was a tracheostomy, an opening in her neck to insert a breathing tube that would connect to a ventilator. She was now six months into life and not even close to eating and breathing like a normal little baby girl, and now operation number four was being proposed — an operation to connect the two ends of her scarred and tethered esophagus.

Mitzi's ICU doctors decreed that if there was ever going to be a good time to try to reattach her esophagus to her stomach, now was the time, before her heart function worsened. This was her window and all she needed was a surgeon.

No one was looking forward to this next chapter. Mitzi was a setup for complications, and every surgeon who had put a knife to her body rediscovered this truth. Suture lines didn't hold. She was a magnet for resistant infections. With no notice at all she would regularly choke, turn blue, and try to die. Operating on Mitzi was like flying over the Bermuda Triangle—the outing might be uneventful, but if it turned into a mysterious series of unexpected horrors, no one would be surprised.

I didn't know if I could repair Mitzi's esophagus any more than the other surgeon who had peered into the mixed-up world of her chest before me. There was no place to pick up spare parts for a baby, although her stomach or small intestine could be repurposed to add length. She was not likely to have a normal life expectancy regardless of whether I was able to reconnect her esophagus, but these complex little patients were famous for proving their doctors wrong. They outlived and outperformed predictions all the time.

Numerous specialists weighed in on Mitzi's condition and what should be done for her next. *Operate now. Wait a few more months. Forget this nonsense and send her to hospice.* Now I had to decide. Did it make sense to operate on Mitzi again, a child with a high operative risk and a limited future, solely to improve her comfort level? Some of my colleagues thought the risk was worth taking. Others thought I was crazy to go down that road, perhaps creating a bigger problem than the ones already at hand. Mitzi might never have a decent quality of life no matter what we did. We were in the gray zone of medical decision making, no right answer and no wrong one either, only instinct and conscience to rely on. Mine told me to give Mitzi her chance.

On the day of Mitzi's operation, a group of nurses came down to the OR with her and took turns playing with her until it was time to go back to the room. They kissed her goodbye and went back upstairs to wait with her toys, blankets, and clothes in the insular world they had created for her.

It took an hour just to prepare Mitzi for the operation, placing IVs and an arterial line for monitoring. Then we set to work. We positioned her on her side and reentered the chest through the incision that had been made before. When we got through to the area where the upper esophagus should have been, there was nothing but dense scar tissue. We couldn't see or feel what we were looking for. I asked the anesthesiologist to insert a large rubber dilator through her mouth into the upper esophagus. He pushed it in and wiggled it around so I could feel it poking just inside the chest. Then I could start dissecting the esophagus out, cutting away the scar tissue as if carving a sculpture out of stone until it started to take shape.

The esophagus was short, stiff, and encased in scar tissue but it was there. Then I pushed on a tube I had inserted through the opening in her stomach, and a little nubbin of lower esophagus came into view. It was thin and the caliber was narrow, but it would be enough to connect to the upper pouch. We were able to draw the two ends close and sew them together using a row of fine sutures placed millimeters apart, front and back. When we were done, I looked at the two ends, one big and bulbous, the other narrow and stretched. It wasn't the prettiest reconstruction, but it had a good chance of healing. We had used every bit of esophagus available. Now we would have to give it a week to heal and perform a barium X-ray to make sure there was no leak.

The hope was that, after her esophagus healed, Mitzi would be able to hold a bottle and drink formula for the first time in her life. Mitzi recovered from her esophageal operation, but after six months of not eating, she had developed an aversion to food. When that happens, it can take weeks to months to get children accustomed to even small feedings. Mitzi got as far as tasting food like popsicles and ice cream, but before she could make much more progress, she developed a severe case of pneumonia and died.

Had we made the right decision for Mitzi? I wouldn't blame anyone for second-guessing her last operation, since she died before she was able to take full feeds by mouth, but as with many other situations in medicine, we couldn't have known before we tried.

The earliest attempts at reconstructing human body parts in the early 1900s used the only thing that was available — a patient's own native tissue. Plastic surgeons were some of the first to utilize a patient's own skin, muscle, and subcutaneous tissue, which could be transposed to various parts of the body to fill in a wound or reconstruct a jaw or a nose. Later, surgeons developed operations that borrowed a portion of the stomach or intestine to aid in the reconstruction of an esophagus removed for cancer or one missing from birth. Intestine has also been used to reconstruct the bladder and vagina.

Synthetic materials, which must be biocompatible (nontoxic to the human body) and durable, were first developed as substitutes for damaged heart valves. In 1952 Hufnagel introduced a Plexiglas cage that could be inserted in place of a faulty aortic valve.[4] This was followed in 1960 by the Sterling Edwards mechanical heart valve, made of plastic, steel, and a cuff of Dacron material used to sew it in place in the heart.[5] Soon afterward, more synthetic materials were introduced, such as the Dacron vascular graft and Teflon tubing, substitutes for obstructed and diseased blood vessels in the upper and lower extremities. Gore-Tex was later produced as tubular conduits to substitute for blood vessels and as sheets that could be configured into a custom patch to close holes in muscular structures throughout the body, such as the heart and diaphragm.

Synthetic materials provided excellent structural support but could not be used as organ substitutes, because they were incapable of performing bodily functions. The intestine, for example, while resembling a simple tube, is lined by microvilli that absorb nutrients. The kidney filters the blood and controls electrolyte balance. The liver, perhaps the most complex organ of all to replicate, manufactures proteins that control blood clotting, metabolizes drugs and toxins, and manufactures bile to aid in digestion.

Until recently, the only conceivable way to replace an organ was to get one from someone else. On the surface, organ transplantation looks like a ready-made solution for babies who are missing parts, but in reality transplantation has not been able to meet the need. There are an estimated 114,000 people in the United States alone on transplant lists waiting for organs, but only 14,000 donated organs per year.[6]

Organ transplantation from human donors began with kidneys in the 1960s and expanded into liver, heart, and lungs over the next twenty years. Small bowel and pancreas transplants have developed over the last decade. To be eligible for a transplant, a candidate must go through a complete physical assessment to determine risk and suitability. Patients are then listed at a particular transplantation center, where they will wait for a suitable, blood type–matched organ. And this is where the enterprise enters the realm of the mercurial, as there is no predicting how long a person might wait. While some organs can be donated from one living person to another—for example, a kidney or a section of liver or lung to a child—organ transplantation is largely dependent on cadaveric donation resulting from human tragedy and the generosity of the aggrieved. Year after year patients who are listed for transplants die before they can receive a lifesaving organ.

While transplanting another human's organs into a person can be lifesaving, there will always be attendant risks, because the tissue of another human being is recognized as foreign by the patient's immune system unless the donor and recipient are identical twins. Because of this, almost all donor transplants require lifelong medication to suppress the immune system to prevent organ rejection. These drugs pose their own set of risks, such as an increased susceptibility to infection and an increased likelihood of cancer later in life. Even after transplant there is a lifelong threat of possible transplant-related complications, such as acute rejection, bleeding, or infection. Organ transplant, therefore, is a lifesaving solution for damaged organs but not a perfect one.

Scientists have known for centuries that the salamander, a distant cousin of the lizard, can grow back a limb when one is lost to the hazards of everyday life. It can also regenerate a tail, a jaw, eyes, and some internal structures. We humans are not so lucky. We cannot grow back our extremities when one gets cut off, although, under some circumstances, we might be able to grow back a fingertip.[7] We can grow back our own skin in limited quantities after a scrape or burn, but only when the wound isn't too large or too deep. Only one human organ, the liver, can truly regenerate— that is, grow back almost entirely—after a portion is surgically removed.

When a limb is amputated, whether salamander or human, cells move into position immediately to seal the wound. Without further intervention, the human body will then lay down layers of fibroblasts that will eventually toughen into a leathery scar. But the salamander cells execute a more creative maneuver: the cells that seal the wound edge will convert to multipotent cells, that is, stem cells that can differentiate in a number of directions and become muscle, skin, bone, and nerve, all the cells that would be required to form a leg. The entire process takes about a month.

Researchers around the world have been trying to tease apart just how the salamander is able to grow back a limb and how it knows exactly how much of it to grow back. For example, if the leg is cut off at the socket, a full-length limb grows back, but if the foot alone is cut off, only that part grows back.

Although scientists have not yet decoded the salamander's special ability to regrow body parts, the field of regenerative medicine has already emerged. This exciting new branch of treatment uses living tissue to repair or replace tissue or body parts that are congenitally absent or have been lost to injury, disease, or aging.[8] Proposed treatments encompass everything from stem cell therapies that stimulate healing, tissue regeneration, and metabolic functions to the creation of implantable tissue-engineered organs.[9]

Dr. Anthony Atala, a pediatric urologist and scientist who has called himself a "reluctant researcher," was spurred into action by his experiences reconstructing children's bladders when he was training in urology. In an operation that had originated during the 1800s, small intestine was used to reconstruct the bladder. The intestine was used because most people had more than they needed and because it could be split down the middle and then sewn back together in the shape of a bladder. But even though the small intestine could be made to look like a bladder, it didn't fully function as one. Complications such as electrolyte abnormalities, excessive mucus production, and mechanical difficulties where the ureters inserted into the bladder were inevitable. The fundamental problem was that the cells lining the intestine, the mucosa, are made to absorb nutrients, whereas the lining of the bladder is designed for excretion.

"Doing bowel-for-bladder replacements in children really got to me," Atala recalled. "It's one thing to put them into an adult, but putting them in a child with a 70-plus life expectancy didn't make sense when you knew there would be trouble down the line."[10]

As Atala became more concerned with the complications of the bladder replacement operation, he began to wonder if it would be possible to grow a new bladder from a patient's own cells. To do so, he would have to learn the basic principles of tissue engineering, a fledgling technique first discovered in the 1970s that had proven capable of generating new cartilage in mice.[11] Skin, cartilage, and bone were some of the first tissues engineered in the laboratory because their structure, compared to that of organs, was relatively simple.

A tissue-engineered organ requires that a scaffold, a three-dimensional replica of the organ, be created first. A scaffold is similar to a framed-in house before the walls and doors are put in. It is constructed of an extracellular matrix that can be created by shaping human- or animal-derived protein from an artificial material such as a type of plastic, or by using a cadaver organ after its native cells are dissolved, leaving just a shell.

The patient's own cells, harvested from a biopsy of their existing native organ mixed with growth factors and other cell nutrients, are sprinkled onto the scaffold and then incubated in a bioreactor, a chamber where bodylike conditions — temperature, humidity, and oxygen concentration — are simulated. Within days to weeks the organ takes shape as tissue grows around and within the scaffold, a process that on time-lapse photography looks like the organ is being spun like cotton candy. Once the organ is fully formed, it is ready to be implanted into the body, where it will be connected to blood vessels and nerves that previously attached to the native organ.

While the concept of building an organ sounds relatively simple in theory, in practice it has taken decades to develop. The bladder, for example — a balloonlike bag that stores urine — is composed of only two cell types, an inner lining and an outer muscle, but it took Atala four years just to grow the cells that could seed a mold in the shape of a bladder and grow successfully into a fully formed bladder.

Three years later, in 1999, he implanted the first laboratory-grown bladder into a child with spina bifida. As reported in 2006, the initial series of seven patients with the first tissue-engineered organs ever implanted into humans did well. Tissue-engineered bladders, derived from a patient's own cells, are currently in clinical trials and will hopefully become commercially available within the next few years.[12]

Tengion, a company cofounded by Atala to commercialize his tissue-engineered inventions, has other first-of-their-kind products in the pipeline, including a "neo-urinary conduit." This is a tissue-engineered substitute for the intestinal diversion of urine many bladder cancer patients require. There is also a "neo-kidney augment" to supplement kidney function while patients are awaiting transplant, a "neo-gastrointestinal augment" for use in esophageal or intestinal disorders, and a "neo-vessel replacement" for use in performing bypasses of coronary or extremity arteries.[13]

Other surgeons have started creating organs in response to a specific clinical need. In the 1980s, pediatric surgeon Dr. Joseph

Vacanti, then in charge of liver transplantation at Boston Children's Hospital, was spurred into action by watching kids get sicker while waiting on the transplant list for an organ. Vacanti partnered with Dr. Robert Langer at MIT to begin what may have been the first laboratory initiative to grow living organs.[14] Their laboratory was the first to produce a lab-grown ear that may soon be implanted into humans. They are also one of the first to produce a beating animal heart and blood vessel tissue and have been working on creating organs with more complex functions, like livers and lungs.[15]

The more complex the function of the organ, the more difficult it is to create, because there are multiple cell types with specialized functions that must be integrated to create a coordinated three-dimensional organ. These more complex organs, like the liver, kidney, and pancreas, are not likely to be available for another ten to twenty years, but the expert consensus is that they will be available eventually.

Meanwhile, news of tissue engineering breakthroughs continues to emerge. In 2012, Dr. Paolo Macchiarini at the Karolinska Institute in Stockholm, Sweden, implanted the first tissue-engineered trachea into a thirty-nine-year-old man.[16] An exact replica of the patient's trachea was made from a porous plastic that was then seeded with stem cells harvested from his bone marrow. The new organ spent only a day and a half in a bioreactor before it was implanted into the patient.

Macchiarini had previously implanted cadaver tracheas that had been reseeded with the intended recipient's own cells into about a dozen patients, most of whom had done well. Preparing a cadaver implant took longer because the original donor cells had to be dissolved from the underlying protein matrix before it could be used. Most intended recipients, pressed by cancer or other life-threatening airway difficulties, were running out of time and desperately needed new tracheas in a shorter time frame. This pushed Macchiarini to shorten the process by producing scaffolds out of plastic. Not only did this technique allow him to make a trachea in just a few days; in addition, because these new implants were custom made, each one was an exact fit.

In 2013, Macchiarini, invited by surgeons at the Children's Hospital of Illinois in Peoria, performed a tracheal implant on a two-year-old who had been born without one, an almost uniformly fatal condition.[17] She was the youngest patient to receive a tissue-engineered organ to date. While she initially appeared to be healing well and adjusting to the new windpipe, three months after the operation she developed a complication and died.[18] This groundbreaking operation, while advancing the cause of tissue-engineered organs one step further, illustrates just how fragile patients who require organ substitutes can be.

The capacity to cure disease and repair anatomic malformations with lab-grown tissue and organs is seemingly unlimited. In addition to the expectation that hearts, livers, kidneys, and gastrointestinal tissue will be available in the coming years, further advances are expected in the treatment of injuries of all kind (including brain and spinal cord) and diseases such as Alzheimer's and diabetes.

Because of the large numbers of wounded soldiers returning from the wars in Iraq and Afghanistan, the military is investing in tissue engineering to speed their recovery. The Armed Forces Institute of Regenerative Medicine (AFIRM) is a network of institutions working toward restoring body parts to injured soldiers and helping them heal wounds with a minimum of scarring and disfigurement.[19] A perfect example of a successful application of regenerative medicine to war wounds is the use of an extracellular protein matrix derived from pigs that is being implanted into injured soldiers to regenerate lost muscle.[20] Once the matrix is implanted into a soldier's wounds, the body starts to break it down as expected, and in the process, the matrix recruits stem cells that will differentiate into muscle cells and restore lost muscle function. The technique, still being refined, has shown promising results.

While tissue engineering has the potential to change the entire landscape of medicine, it will also open up new areas of controversy. How much of a person can or should be rebuilt? Will there be any long-term health consequences to tissue engineering, such as cells leaching out of implanted organs and becoming renegade cancerous masses in some other part of the body? Will implanting homegrown organs be more or less costly than organ transplantation? What are the limits to tissue engineering—for example, will we be able to grow every organ in the body, even a human brain? Will there be an impetus to completely regenerate a human being, to preserve a person's brain and deposit it in an entirely new body? Ethical issues associated with tissue-engineered organs will have to be addressed just as similar issues were addressed when organ transplantation was introduced.

In the meantime, the way we treat babies who are born without organs or who lose them to life-threatening diseases is bound to change. Since the inception of the field, pediatric surgeons have struggled with replacing body parts in children, borrowing tissue from other structures in the body to replace what was missing, sometimes taking kids back to the operating room for multiple operations in a sequence of step-by-step maneuvers to reconstruct missing organs. In the next decade pediatric surgery will be transformed as a result of advances in creating new biomaterials and tissue engineered body parts.

We are on the verge of an era where the technology will exist to implant bioengineered organs either in utero or shortly after birth. Babies facing certain death in the past, like the majority of those discussed in the preceding chapters, will have options that will virtually guarantee survival. Babies born with severe intestinal atresias, like Baby K. who did not survive in the 1960s, will be rescued from short gut syndrome with intestinal conduits grown from their own stem cells. When a baby is born with a hole in his diaphragm, like Baby X., not only will the hole be patched with muscular tissue that can grow with him, but also perhaps a new set of lungs can be implanted—if the lungs haven't already been salvaged with an in utero procedure.

One can imagine that a baby missing an intact esophagus, like Mitzi, will have a new one grown in the lab, the perfect size for implantation after she is born. Or projecting further into the future, in what might sound like science fiction to us today, before a baby like Mitzi is even born, the seeds for a fully formed esophagus could be implanted by injecting stem cells in utero and training them to grow on a scaffold like a trumpet vine on a trellis. And we might be able to create a new heart for her too if she needs it—a chance to begin life with all the missing parts replaced with organs that will grow with her into the future.

The next generation of replacement organs will also offer hope to children who are the victims of childhood cancer. Currently, if a tumor has extended into a vital organ it may not be possible to remove it, but if tissue-engineered replacements are readily available, the entire therapeutic landscape for kidney, lung, and liver tumors will be transformed. Physicians will be able to regenerate bone tissue to fill in limbs rather than performing amputations. Victims of traumatic injury will likewise benefit from the capability to remove damaged organs and replace them with healthy ones.

It's difficult to know how the barrage of advances in prenatal diagnosis, fetal surgery, precision instruments and devices engineered for the pediatric market, and tissue-engineered organs will mesh in the coming decades. There will still be times when a surgeon will need to have heart-wrenching conversations with stunned parents because she cannot save an infant, but one hopes that within the next decade these conversations will become less frequent as the landscape for replacement parts transforms the practice of pediatric surgery.

Will the future be any more amazing than the first sixty years of pediatric surgery, when our predecessors created a specialty devoted to repairing tiny body parts using tools and techniques they crafted themselves? Such a scenario seems difficult to imagine, but the answer is on the horizon.

acknowledgments

Pediatric surgeons get to work with two never-ending sources of inspiration — kids, who live for today and remind us that having fun should be a priority, and their parents, who continually show us, especially when a child is in the hospital, that there are no limits to the power of love. I am grateful to both for their smiles and hugs and for the courage they show in the face of grave circumstances.

This book began as a series of scribbles in a journal late at night, a way to unwind after long days in the hospital. My amazing agent, Laurie Abkemier, found a way to turn these rambling tales into a book. Without her, there would be no *Small*. Laurie's hard work led me to Stephen Hull, my editor at the University Press of New England. Steve and I immediately bonded through our mutual love of sports and the stories in *Small*. I appreciate the generous patience and support that both showed in dealing with a first-time author.

Many heroes make appearances in this book — surgeons, mentors, parents, and patients. I am especially grateful to Dr. Stan Dudrick, Dr. Barbara Barlow, and Dr. James Fischer for sharing their contributions to the field of pediatric surgery and helping me bring them to life. Dr. Barlow, Dr. Ann Kosloske, and Dr. Carmen Ramos reviewed the manuscript for accuracy and provided numerous insights.

I thank Spike Gillespie, who read the first spiral-bound version of *Small* in her bathtub, making notes in the margin as she turned the damp pages. Her early belief in the project helped propel it to completion. Shelley Austin taught me how queries, agents, and publishers worked and wrote my first query letter. Beth Moten provided me with the company of three hundred head of Charlemagne cattle and a quiet place to write at the Moten Ranch.

I am especially grateful to Anne Morgan — my first reader, my last reader, the person who would never let me quit.

Catherine Musemeche

1. the thread of life

1 Thomas W. Sadler, *Langman's Medical Embryology* (Baltimore: Lippincott, Williams & Wilkins, 2012), 63.

2 S. E. Parker, C. T. Mai, M. A. Canfield, et al., for the National Birth Defects Prevention Network, "Updated National Birth Prevalence Estimates for Selected Birth Defects in the United States, 2004–2006," *Birth Defects Research Part A: Clinical and Molecular Teratology* (2010), http://www.cdc.gov/ncbddd/features /birthdefects-keyfindings.html.

3 J. Petrini, K. Damus, R. Russell, K. Poschman, M. J. Davidoff, and D. Mattison, "Contribution of Birth Defects to Infant Mortality in the United States," *Teratology* 66 (2002): 3–6, http://www.ncbi.nlm .nih.gov/pubmed/12239736.

4 Sadler, *Langman's Medical Embryology*, 13.

5 Ibid.

6 G. H. Valentine, "Incidence of Chromosome Disorders," *Canadian Family Physician* 25 (1979): 938.

7 Alok Sharma, Simon Ford, and Jennifer Calvert, "Adaptation for Life: A Review of Neonatal Physiology," *Anaesthesia and Intensive Care Medicine* 12 (2010): 85–90.

8 Sadler, *Langman's Medical Embryology*, 217.

9 Ibid., 227.

2. bunny rabbits, boston, and babies

1 Willis J. Potts, "Pediatric Surgery," *Journal of the American Medical Association* 157 (1955): 629.

2 Robert E. Gross, *The Surgery of Infancy and Childhood: Its Principles and Techniques* (Philadelphia: W. B. Saunders, 1953), 26–29.

3 A. M. Rivera, K. W. Strauss, A. van Zundert, and E. Mortier, "The History of Peripheral Intravenous Catheters: How Little Plastic

Tubes Revolutionized Medicine," *Acta Anaesthesiologica Belgica* 56 (2005): 277.

4 C. Everett Koop, "A Perspective on the Early Days of Pediatric Surgery," *Journal of Pediatric Surgery* 34 (1999): 41. "The technique of administering fluids in those days was abysmal," Koop wrote. One of his own children became dehydrated and was treated with a "clysis of saline injected under the skin between his scapulae. He had a 'tumor' on his back as big as a grapefruit."

5 C. Everett Koop, *Koop: The Memoirs of America's Family Doctor* (Grand Rapids: Zondervan, 1992), 105.

6 Ibid.

7 Ibid., 101.

8 Ibid.

9 Ibid.

10 John G. Raffensperger, *Children's Surgery: A Worldwide History* (Jefferson, NC: McFarland & Co., 2012), 115.

11 Ibid.

12 Ibid.

13 Jason C. Fisher, Mark A. Hardy, and Warren D. Widmann, "Robert E. Gross: The Heart of a Surgeon," *Current Surgery* 62 (2005): 496.

14 Ibid., 497.

15 J. Alex Haller, "Why Pediatric Surgery? A Personal Journey through the First 50 Years," *Annals of Surgery* 237 (2003): 597–606, quotation 597, http://www.ncbi.nlm.nih.gov/pmc/articles /PMC1514508.

16 Ibid.

17 Koop, "A Perspective on the Early Days of Pediatric Surgery," 40.

18 Haller, "Why Pediatric Surgery?," 598.

19 Potts, "Pediatric Surgery," 627.

20 Ibid., 628.

21 Koop, "A Perspective on the Early Days of Pediatric Surgery," 42; Haller, "Why Pediatric Surgery?," 598.

22 Koop, "A Perspective on the Early Days of Pediatric Surgery," 41.

23 Koop, *Koop*, 128.

24 Selma H. Calmes, "The First Anesthesiologist at America's First Children's Hospital: Margo Deming, M.D. (1914–1998) and the Children's Hospital of Philadelphia," *American Society of*

Anesthesiology Newsletter 62 (1998): 1, http://anestit.unipa.it
/mirror/asa2/newsletters/1998/10_98/First_1098.html (accessed
January 16, 2014).

25 Ibid., 2.

26 Koop, "A Perspective on the Early Days of Pediatric Surgery," 43.

27 Associated Press, "Kennedy Infant Dies at Boston Hospital;
President at Hand," *New York Times*, August 9, 1963.

28 Sylvia Wrobel, "Bubbles, Babies and Biology: The Story of
Surfactant," *FASEB Journal* 18 (2004): 1, http://www.fasebj.org
/content/18/13/1624e.full.

29 Peter A. Southorn and Bradley J. Narr, "The Massa or Rochester
Plastic Needle," *Mayo Clinic Proceedings* 83 (2008): 1165.

30 Ibid.

31 Rivera et al., "The History of Peripheral Intravenous Catheters," 276.

32 Koop, "A Perspective on the Early Days of Pediatric Surgery," 43.

33 Haller, "Why Pediatric Surgery?," 601.

3. the shortcut to survival

1 Douglas W. Wilmore and Stanley J. Dudrick, "Growth and
Development of an Infant Receiving All Nutrients Exclusively by
Vein," *Journal of the American Medical Association* 203 (1968): 140.

2 Wolfgang F. Caspary, "Physiology and Pathophysiology of Intestinal
Absorption," *American Journal of Clinical Nutrition* 55 (1992):
299S–307S.

3 Ibid.

4 Carmen Cuffari, "Pediatric Short Bowel Syndrome," http://
emedicine.medscape.com/article/931855-overview (accessed
November 10, 2013).

5 Stanley J. Dudrick, "History of Parenteral Nutrition," in an address
to the annual meeting of the American College of Nutrition,
October 1, 2009, Orlando, FL, http://www.jacn.org/conent/28/3
/243.full, p. 10.

6 George W. Holcomb and J. P. Murphy, eds., *Ashcraft's Pediatric
Surgery* (Philadelphia: Saunders, Elsevier, 2010), 19–23.

7 Stanley J. Dudrick, MD, Oral History Project interview, Pediatric
History Center (Elk Grove Village, IL: American Academy of
Pediatrics, 2007), 24.

8 Ibid., 31.
9 Dudrick, "History of Parenteral Nutrition," 10.
10 Dudrick, Oral History Project interview, 32.
11 45 CFR § 46, Subpart A: Basic HHS Policy for Protection of Human Research Subjects, http://www.hhs.gov/ohrp/human subjects/guidance/45cfr46.html (accessed February 2, 2013).
12 Dudrick, Oral History Project interview, 32.
13 Wilmore and Dudrick, "Growth and Development of an Infant," 142.
14 Dudrick, "History of Parenteral Nutrition," 2.
15 Dudrick, Oral History Project interview, 35–36.
16 Dudrick, "History of Parenteral Nutrition," 10.

4. inside out

1 Raffensperger, Children's Surgery, 217.
2 Ibid., 218.
3 S. R. Schuster, "A New Method for the Staged Repair of Large Omphaloceles," Surgery, Gynecology and Obstetrics 125 (1967): 837–850.
4 Raffensperger, Children's Surgery, 231.
5 Personal communication (email) from James Fischer, MD, to the author, January 26, 2013.

5. going to extremes

1 Robert H. Bartlett, "Surgery, Science and Respiratory Failure," Journal of Pediatric Surgery 32 (1997): 1402.
2 Adora Ann Fou, "John H. Gibbon: The First 20 Years of the Heart-Lung Machine," Texas Heart Institute Journal 24 (1997): 1–2.
3 Ibid.
4 William S. Stoney, "Historical Perspectives in Cardiology: Evolution of Cardiopulmonary Bypass," Circulation 119 (2009): 2847.
5 Ibid.
6 Fou, "John H. Gibbon," 1–2.
7 Stoney, "Historical Perspectives in Cardiology," 2844–2853.
8 Ibid.
9 Ibid.
10 Ibid.

11 Bartlett, "Surgery, Science and Respiratory Failure," 1403.

12 Ibid.

13 Extracorporeal Life Support Organization, Ann Arbor, "ECLS Registry Report, International Summary, July, 2012," http://www .elsonet.org/index.php/registry/statistics/limited.html (accessed January 23, 2013).

14 Heidi J. Dalton, Peter T. Rycus, and Steven A. Conrad, "Update on Extracorporeal Life Support 2004," *Seminars in Perinatology* (2005): 24.

6. battlegrounds to playgrounds

1 Barbara Barlow, MD, interviewed April 10, 2008, by Suzanne Boulter, MD, in New York, NY, for the Oral History Project, Pediatric History Center (American Academy of Pediatrics, Elk Grove Village, IL, 2007), 24. Further details of Dr. Barlow's experiences at Harlem Hospital were conveyed via personal communications (emails) with the author, February–March 2013.

2 Michael Sterne, "In the Last Decade, Leaders Say, Harlem's Dreams Have Died," *New York Times*, March 1, 1978.

3 http://www.cdc.gov/injury/index.html (accessed September 29, 2013).

4 Daniel M. Alterman, "Considerations in Pediatric Trauma," *Medscape*, http://emedicine.medscape.com/article/435031-overview #aw2aab6b3 (accessed January 18, 2013).

5 Barlow, Oral History Project interview, 1.

6 Nancy Groves, "From Past to Present: the Changing Demographics of Women in Medicine," http://www.aao.org/yo/newsletter/200806 /article04.cfm (accessed January 26, 2013).

7 Barlow, Oral History Project interview, 6.

8 Ibid.

9 Ibid.

10 Philip L. Glick and Richard G. Azizkhan, *A Genealogy of North American Pediatric Surgery: From Ladd until Now* (St. Louis: Quality Medical Publishing, 1997), 6–138. The number of officially trained pediatric surgeons from 1937 to 1973 was tabulated from charts that reconstructed the genealogy of pediatric surgery training programs.

11 Juliet A. Emamaullee, Megan V. Lyons, Elizabeth Berdan, and Amy

Bazzarelli, "Women Leaders in Surgery: Past, Present, and Future," *Bulletin of the American College of Surgeons* 97 (2012): 24–29, quotation on 25.

12 Barlow, Oral History Project interview, 25.

13 David C. Grossman, "The History of Injury Control and the Epidemiology of Child and Adolescent Injuries," *Future of Children* 10 (2000): 23–52, quotation on 25.

14 Ibid.

15 National Highway Traffic Safety Administration, *Traffic Safety Facts: Occupant Protection*, Data. Pub. No. DOT HS 811 160 (2008), http://www-nrd.nhtsa.dot.gov/Pubs/811160.pdf (accessed February 1, 2013).

16 Robert W. Stock, "Safety Lessons from the Morgue," *New York Times*, October 26, 2012, http://www.nytimes.com/2012/10/28 /magazine/safety-lessons-from-the-morgue.html.

17 Susan P. Baker, *Fifty Favorites from the Works of Susan P. Baker* (Baltimore: Johns Hopkins Center for Injury Research and Policy, 2012), 1–63, quotation on 53.

18 Douglas Martin, "About New York," *New York Times*, July 20, 1991, http://www.nytimes.com/1991/07/20/nyregion/about-new-york .html.

19 "About the Injury Free Coalition for Kids," http://www.injuryfree .org/about_history.cfm (accessed February 2, 2013).

20 Centers for Disease Control, *Saving Lives and Protecting People from Violence and Injury*, http://www.cdc.gov/injury/overview/index.html (accessed January 31, 2013).

21 "CDC Foundation Hero Award," http://www.cdcfoundation.org /what/program/cdc-foundation-hero-award (accessed February 2, 2013).

22 David Hemenway, *While We Were Sleeping: Success Stories in Injury and Violence Prevention* (Berkeley: University of California Press, 2009), 82.

7. the weight of the future

1 Centers for Disease Control and Prevention, "Childhood Obesity Facts," http://www.cdc.gov/healthyyouth/obesity/facts.htm (accessed February 11, 2013).

2 Robert Wood Johnson Foundation, "Declining Childhood Obesity Rates — Where Are We Seeing the Most Progress?," Issue Brief, September 2012, http://www.rwjf.org/content/dam/farm/reports /issue_briefs/2012/rwjf401163.

3 Jan Hoffman, "A Child's Helping Hand on Portions," *New York Times*, April 24, 2012, http://www.nytimes.com/2012/04/25/dining /a-child-offers-plan-on-portion-control-for-dieters.htm.

4 BMI, or body mass index, takes into consideration a person's height and weight and is therefore considered a more reliable indicator than weight alone of whether a person is overweight or obese (18.5– 25 = normal, 25–30 = overweight, > 30 = obese); see http://www .cdc.gov/healthyweight/assessing/bmi/ (accessed May 24, 2013).

5 Hoffman, "A Child's Helping Hand on Portions."

6 Kelly D. Brownell, "Thinking Forward: The Quicksand of Appeasing the Food Industry," *PLoS Med* 9 (2012), http://www .plosmedicine.org/article/info%3Adoi%2F10.1371%2Fjournal.pmed .1001254 (accessed February 10, 2013).

7 Michael Moss, "The Extraordinary Science of Junk Food," *New York Times Magazine*, February 20, 2013, http://www.nytimes.com/2013 /02/24/magazine/the-extraordinary-science-of-junk-food.htm.

8 Jeffrey Levi, Laura M. Segal, Rebecca St. Laurent, and David Kohn, *F as in Fat 2011: How Obesity Threatens America's Future* (Trust for America's Health and the Robert Wood Johnson Foundation, July 2011), http://www.rwjf.org/en/research-publications/find-rwjf -research/2011/07/f-as-in-fat.htm.

9 Kelly Brownell, "Let's Get Real: The Portion War between Big Soda and NYC Is All about Profit," *The Atlantic*, June 15, 2012, http:// www.theatlantic.com/health/archive/2012/06/lets-get-real-the -portion-war-between-big-soda-and-nyc-is-all-about-profit/258546/.

10 John Cawley and Chad Meyerhoefer, "The Medical Costs of Obesity: An Instrumental Variables Approach," *Journal of Health Economics* 31 (2012): 219–230.

11 Levi et al., *F as in Fat 2011*.

12 Rebecca M. Puhl and Chelsea A. Heuer, "The Stigma of Obesity: A Review and Update," *Obesity* (2009), http://www.yaleruddcenter .org/resources/upload/docs/what/bias/WeightBiasStudy.pdf (accessed February 18, 2013).

13   The Rudd Center, "Sugar-Sweetened Beverages Fact Sheet:
     Avoiding Weight Bias in Portrayals of Overweight and Obese
     People in Media Campaigns," http://yaleruddcenter.org/resources
     /upload/docs/what/policy/SSBtaxes/SSB_MediaStigma_Fa112010
     (accessed January 16, 2014,); Chelsea A. Heuer, " 'Fattertainment':
     Obesity in the Media," http://www.obesityaction.org/educational
     -resources/resource-articles-2/weight-bias/fattertainment-obesity
     -in-the-media (accessed March 7, 2013).

14   Ibid.

15   http://www.obesityaction.org/ (accessed January 16, 2014).

16   Richard S. Nelson, Robert Kolts, Roger Park, et al., "A Comparison
     of Cholecystectomy and Observation in Children with Biliary
     Dyskinesia," *Journal of Pediatric Surgery* 41 (2006): 1897.

17   "The Big Mac Index," *The Economist*, December 15, 2012, http://
     www.economist.com/news/special-report/21568068-burger
     -company-may-be-barometer-industry-big-mac-index.

18   Anthony Ramirez, "Fast Food Lightens Up but Sales Are Often
     Thin," *New York Times*, March 19, 1991, http://www.nytimes.com
     /1991/03/19/business/fast-food-lightens-up-but-sales-are-often-thin
     .html?pagewanted=all&src=pm.

19   Roberta R. Friedman and Kelly D. Brownell / Yale Rudd Center
     for Policy and Obesity, "Rudd Report: Sugar-Sweetened Beverage
     Taxes," October 2012, http://www.yaleruddcenter.org. SSBs
     are defined as "any beverage with added sugar or other caloric
     sweeteners such as high fructose corn syrup, including soda,
     sports drinks, fruit drinks, teas, flavored waters and energy
     drinks."

20   FDA Consumer Health Information / US Food and Drug
     Administration, "FDA Targets Trans Fat in Processed Food,"
     November 2013, http://www.fda.gov/downloads/ForConsumers
     /ConsumerUpdates/UCM373957.pdf.

21   Julie Jargon, "Low-Cal Items Fuel Restaurant Sales," *Wall Street
     Journal*, February 7, 2013, http://online.wsj.com/article/SB10001424
     127887324906004578288301394995968.html.

22   Alexandra Sifferlin, "Childhood Obesity Rates Drop Slightly in
     Some Cities: What Are They Doing Right," *Time*, December 12,

2012, http://healthland.time.com/2012/12/12/childhood-obesity
-rates-drop-slightly-in-some-cities-what-are-they-doing-right.

23 Anemona Hartocollis, "Young, Obese and in Surgery," *New York Times*, January 7, 2012, http://www.nytimes.com/2012/01/08/health /young-obese-and-getting-weight-loss-surgery.html.

24 Lauren Marcus and Amanda Baron, "Childhood Obesity: The Effects on Physical and Mental Health," http://www.aboutourkids .org/articles/childhood_obesity_effects_physical_mental_health (accessed October 3, 2013).

25 Paul E. O'Brien, Susan M. Sawyer, Cheryl Laurie, et al., "Laparoscopic Adjustable Gastric Banding in Severely Obese Adolescents," *Journal of the American Medical Association*, February 10, 2010, http://jama.jamanetwork.com/article.aspx?articleid =185355. O'Brien et al. found that, in a clinical trial comparing weight loss success in adolescents undergoing gastric banding versus lifestyle intervention, 84 percent in the gastric banding versus 12 percent in the lifestyle group lost more than 50 percent of excess weight.

26 International Pediatric Endosurgery Group (IPEG), "Guidelines for Surgical Treatment of Clinically Severely Obese Adolescents," http://www.ipeg.org/morbidobesity/ (accessed January 16, 2014).

8. something to celebrate

1 Fact Sheet on Childhood Cancers, the National Cancer Institute (2008), http://www.cancer.gov/cancertopics/factsheet/Sites-Types /childhood (accessed March 11, 2013).

2 George W. Holcombe III and J. Patrick Murphy, eds., *Ashcraft's Pediatric Surgery*, 5th ed. (Philadelphia: Saunders, 2010), 838.

3 Ira Flatow, "The War on Cancer Turns 40," *Science Times* on NPR, December 23, 2011, http://www.npr.org/2011/12/23/144190091/the -war-on-cancer-turns-40.

4 "Cancer Facts and the War on Cancer," http://training.seer.cancer .gov/disease/war/ (accessed March 31, 2013).

5 "Cancer Death Rates Drop Significantly," *Medical News Today*, http://www.medicalnewstoday.com/articles/255192.php (accessed March 31, 2013).

6 Denis R. Miller, "A Tribute to Sidney Farber—the Father of Modern Chemotherapy," *British Journal of Haematology* 134 (2006): 20–26, http://onlinelibrary.wiley.com/doi/10.1111/j.1365-2141.2006 .06119.x/full.

7 Ibid.

8 Ibid.

9 Ibid.

10 Ann C. Mertens, Yutaka Yasui, Joseph P. Neglia, et al., "Late Mortality Experience in Five-Year Survivors of Childhood and Adolescent Cancer: The Childhood Cancer Survivor Study," *Journal of Clinical Oncology* 19 (2001): 3163–3172, http://jco.ascopubs.org /content/19/13/3163.full.pdf.

11 Don Norwood, "Pediatric and Adult Cancer Patients Face Different Issues in Care, Survivorship," *Oncolog* 57 (2012), http://www2 .mdanderson.org/depts/oncolog/articles/12/2-feb/2-12-1.html.

12 Kevin C. Oeffinger, Ann C. Mertens, Charles A. Sklar, et al., "Chronic Health Conditions in Adult Survivors of Childhood Cancer," *New England Journal of Medicine* 355 (2006): 1572–1582, http://live.childrens.com/Assets/Documents/specialties /AftertheCancerExperience(ACE)/NEJM2006article.pdf.

9. tiny tools for tiny bodies

1 Tom Pedulla, "Back from War, Columbia Slugger Is Dreaming of the Major Leagues," *New York Times*, May 20, 2013.

2 "The Titanium Rib," *Moving Stories: 75 Years of Orthopaedics*, http:// www.aaos75th.org/stories/physician_story.htm?id=15 (accessed May 7, 2013).

3 Ibid.

4 John Seabrook, *Flash of Genius and Other True Stories of Invention* (New York: St. Martin's Griffin, 2008), 1.

5 Ibid., 13–31. Kearns shared his design for the intermittent wiper with automakers who declined to license his patented invention. When the intermittent wiper started turning up on vehicles, Kearns took them apart and found a design very similar to his own. After lengthy legal proceedings he successfully sued Ford, GM, and Chrysler for patent infringement.

6   "Know How: Thomas Fogarty," http://www.mit.edu/~invent/ima
    /fogarty_bio.html (accessed October 14, 2013).

7   "What's the Master Medical Device Maker's Secret?," *Stanford
    Medicine Magazine*, Fall 2006, http://stanmed.stanford.edu
    /2006fall/fogarty.html.

8   Ibid.

9   "A Fireside Chat with the 'Edison of Medicine,' Thomas Fogarty,
    MD," Fogarty Institute for Innovation (videotaped interview
    conducted by Brian Buntz), http://www.fogartyinstitute.org/news
    -20120420.html (accessed October 15, 2013).

10 Ibid.

11 "What's the Master Medical Device Maker's Secret?"

12 "A Fireside Chat with the 'Edison of Medicine,' Thomas Fogarty,
    MD."

13 Fogarty Institute for Innovation, http://www.fogartyinstitute.org
    /about.html (accessed October 15, 2013).

14 The FDA divides medical devices into three classes based on
    the risk: Class I devices are low-risk devices such as bandages
    or tongue depressors. Class II devices might include tools used
    inside the body. Class III devices are those with greatest risk, e.g.,
    implantable devices such as pacemakers.

15 US Department of Health and Human Services, Food and Drug
    Administration, "Innovation or Stagnation: Challenge and
    Opportunity on the Critical Path to New Medical Products," March
    2004, http://www.nipte.org/docs/Critical_Path.pdf.

16 Will Sansom, "Titanium Triumph: Reinventing the Rib," *Mission*,
    November 2004, . http://uthscsa.edu/mission/article.asp?id=283.

17 "The Titanium Rib."

18 Sansom, "Titanium Triumph."

19 "The Titanium Rib Project," http://www.uthscsa.edu/hscnews/pdf
    /TitaniumRibProject.pdf (accessed January 16, 2014).

20 US Government Accountability Office, "Pediatric Medical Devices:
    Provisions Support Development, but Better Data Needed for
    Required Reporting," December 2011: GAo–12–225, 6, http://www
    .gao.gov/products/GAO-12–225. According to the FDA, medical
    devices include "items used for the diagnosis, cure, mitigation,

treatment, or prevention of a disease" and may range from a bandage to a surgical tool to a pacemaker.

21 "Children as a Percentage of the Population: Persons in Selected Age Groups as a Percentage of the Total U.S. Population, and Children Ages 0–17 as a Percentage of the Dependent Population, 1950–2011 and Projected 2012–2050," http://www.childstats.gov /americaschildren/tables/pop2.asp (accessed May 5, 2013). The 0–17 population peaked from 1960 to 1966 at 36 percent and has been steadily dropping ever since. By 2050 it will be down to 23 percent.

22 Laurie Tarkan, "Medical Devices Fall Short for Children," *New York Times*, May 6, 2013.

23 "Pediatric Medical Devices: Provisions Support Development, but Better Data Needed for Required Reporting," 14.

24 Tarkan, "Medical Devices Fall Short for Children."

25 "Office of Orphan Products Development," US Food and Drug Administration, http://www.fda.gov/AboutFDA/CentersOffices /OfficeofMedicalProductsandTobacco/OfficeofScienceandHealth Coordination/ucm2018190.htm (accessed May 10, 2013).

26 "The Titanium Rib Project," http://www.uthscsa.edu/hscnews/pdf /TitaniumRibProject.pdf (accessed May 28, 2013).

27 Pediatric Device Consortia Grant Program (P50), Department of Health and Human Services, http://grants.nih.gov/grants/guide/rfa -files/RFA-FD-13–010.html (accessed January 16, 2014).

28 Multicenter Trial for Magnetic Mini-Mover for Pectus Excavatum (3MP), http://clinicaltrials.gov/ct2/show/NCT01327274 (accessed January 18, 2014).

29 Michael Harrison, et al., "Magnetic Mini-Mover Procedure for Pectus Excavatum II: Initial Findings of a Food and Drug Administration–Sponsored Trial," *Journal of Pediatric Surgery* 45 (2010): 185–191.

30 Jenny Blair, "Printing's Next Dimension," *Alcalde*, March/April 2013, 22.

31 Jeff Swiatek, "Cook Medical Method Fixes Blocked Glands," April 4, 2013, WBNS 10-TV, http://www.10tv.com/content/stories /apexchange/2013/04/04/in--exchange-salivary-gland-treatment .html.

32 Phil Sneiderman, "Johns Hopkins Team Deploys Hundreds of
Tiny Untethered Surgical Tools in First Animal Biopsies," Johns
Hopkins University News Release, April 23, 2013, http://releases
.jhu.edu/2013/04/23/johns-hopkins-team-deploys-hundreds-of-tiny
-untethered-surgical-tools-in-first-animal-biopsies/.

10. lessons

1 "To Err Is Human: Building a Safer Health System," Institute of
Medicine, November 1999, http://www.iom.edu/Reports/1999/to
-err-is-human-building-a-safer-health-system.aspx. Not all jumbo
jetliners have the same passenger capacity. Using a figure of 98,000
deaths per year, a Boeing 787 Dreamliner, with a capacity of 250–
290 patients, is the most accurate for comparison. See "Boeing
Dreamliner 787, Airbus A380 and the Jumbo Jet: How Do They
Compare?," http://www.telegraph.co.uk/travel/travelnews/9221338
/Boeing-Dreamliner-787-Airbus-A380-and-the-jumbo-jet-How-do
-they-compare.html (accessed November 16, 2013).

2 Marty Makary, "How to Stop Hospitals from Killing Us," *Wall Street
Journal*, September 21, 2012, http://online.wsj.com/news/articles
/SB10000872396390444620104578008263334441352.

3 Marshall Allen, "How Many Die from Mistakes in U.S. Hospitals?,"
ProPublica, September 19, 2013, http://www.propublica.org/article
/how-many-die-from-medical-mistakes-in-us-hospitals.

4 "Feds Extend Pilots' Rest Time to Avoid Fatigue," *CBS News Online*,
December 21, 2011, http://www.cbsnews.com/8301-201_162
-57346125/feds-extend-pilots-rest-time-to-avoid-fatigue/.

5 Ibid.

6 Ibid.

7 Barron H. Lerner, "A Life-Changing Case for Doctors in Training,"
New York Times, March 3, 2009, http://www.nytimes.com/2009/03
/03/health/03zion.html.

8 Ibid.

9 Ibid.

10 Christopher P. Landrigan, Jeffrey M. Rothschild, John W. Cronin,
et al., "Effect of Reducing Interns' Work Hours on Serious Medical
Errors in Intensive Care Units," *New England Journal of Medicine* 351
(2004): 1838.

11 Darshak Sanghavi, "The Phantom Menace of Sleep-Deprived Doctors," *New York Times*, August 5, 2011, http://www.nytimes.com /2011/08/07/magazine/the-phantom-menace-of-sleep-deprived -doctors.html.

12 Ibid.

13 Jeffery M. Rothschild, Carol A. Keohane, Selwyn Rogers, et al., "Risks of Complications by Attending Physicians after Performing Nighttime Procedures," *Journal of the American Medical Association* 302 (2009): 1565–1572, http://jama.jamanetwork.com/article.aspx ?articleid=184705.

14 Maggie Jones, "How Little Sleep Can You Get Away With?," *New York Times*, April 15, 2011, http://www.nytimes.com/2011/04/17 /magazine/mag-17Sleep-t.html.

15 Michael J. Breus, "Sleep Habits: More Important Than You Think," *WebMD*, http://www.webmd.com/sleep-disorders/features /important-sleep-habits.

16 Ibid.

17 Lulu Xie, Hongyi Kang, Qiwu Xu, et al., "Sleep Drives Metabolite Clearance from the Adult Brain," *Science* 18 (2013): 373–377.

11. small

1 Tim Jancelewicz and Michael R. Harrison, "A History of Fetal Surgery," *Clinics in Perinatology* 36 (2009): 229.

2 Margaret B. McNay and John E. E. Fleming, "Forty Years of Obstetric Ultrasound 1957–1997: From A-Scope to Three Dimensions," *Ultrasound in Medicine and Biology* 25 (1999): 45.

3 Jancelewicz and Harrison, "A History of Fetal Surgery," 230.

4 Juliana Bunim, "UCSF Surgeon Reflects on Performing World's First Fetal Surgery 30 Years Ago," http://www.ucsf.edu/news/2011 /02/9366/ucsf-surgeon-reflects-performing-worlds-first-fetal -surgery-30-years-ago.

5 Michael R. Harrison, et al., *The Unborn Patient: The Art and Science of Fetal Therapy*, 3rd ed. (New York: Saunders, 2001).

6 "Doctors Skeptical of Fetal Surgery," *Spokane Chronicle*, July 31, 1986, 1.

7 Sadler, *Langman's Medical Embryology*, 96–99.

8 Sabin Russell, "First Fetal Surgery Survivor Finally Meets His

Doctor: 24 Years Ago, UCSF Surgeon Saved His Life in Mom's Womb," *San Francisco Chronicle*, May 5, 2005, http://www.sfgate .com/health/article/SAN-FRANCISCO-First-fetal-surgery-survivor -2348923.php.

9 Ibid.

10 Michael Harrison et al., "A Randomized Trial of Fetal Endoscopic Tracheal Occlusion for Severe Fetal Congenital Diaphragmatic Hernia," *New England Journal of Medicine* 349 (2003): 1916–1924.

11 Margaret B. McNay and John E. E. Fleming, "Forty Years of Obstetric Ultrasound, 1957–1997: From A-Scope to Three Dimensions," *Ultrasound in Medicine and Biology* 25 (1999): 3–56, quotation on 6.

12 Ibid., 8.

13 Ibid., 10.

14 Ibid., 47.

15 Alan W. Flake, "Surgery in the Human Fetus: The Future," *Journal of Physiology* 15 (2003): 45–51, http://www.ncbi.nlm.nih.gov/pmc /articles/PMC2342614.

16 N. S. Adzick, E. A. Thom, C. Y. Spong, et al., "A Randomized Trial of Prenatal versus Postnatal Repair of Myelomeningocele," *New England Journal of Medicine* 364 (2011): 993–1004.

17 Shinjiro Hirose, Diana L. Farmer, Hanmin Lee, et al., "The Ex Utero Intrapartum Treatment Procedure: Looking Back at the EXIT," *Journal of Pediatric Surgery* 39 (2003): 375–380.

18 Michael R. Harrison, "Fetal Surgery," *Western Journal of Medicine* 159 (1993): 341–349.

19 Daniel Costello, "Too Much Risk?," *Los Angeles Times*, September 26, 2005, http://articles.latimes.com/2005/sep/26/health/he -feta126 (stating that there is no national registry for fetal surgeries, so no one knows exactly how many procedures are done per year or the outcomes from such procedures).

20 Leslie Hill, "Fetal Surgery's Benefits Need Further Study: Report," *Reporter: Vanderbilt University Medical Center's Weekly Newspaper*, April 7, 2011, http://www.mc.vanderbilt.edu/reporter/index.html ?ID=10510.

21 Michael R. Harrison, "Fetal Surgery: Trial, Tribulations and Turf," *Journal of Pediatric Surgery* 38 (2003): 272–282.

12. the lost and found

1 *Robert E. Gross, The Surgery of Infancy and Childhood* (Philadelphia: W. B. Saunders, 1953), 83.

2 Ibid., 81.

3 Ibid., 82.

4 D. Jaron, P. Lelkes, R. Seliktar, et al., "Mechanical Heart Valve," http://www.pages.drexel.edu/~nag38/Materials.html (accessed November 13, 2013).

5 Ibid.

6 Ed Yong, "Replacement Parts," *The Scientist*, August 1, 2012, http:// www.the-scientist.com/?articles.view/articleNo/32409/title /Replacement-Parts/.

7 "Fingertip Injuries and Amputations," http://orthoinfo.aaos.org /topic.cfm?topic=A00014 (accessed May 28, 2013). Fingertips, particularly in patients under the age of two, have also reportedly grown back in entirety in some patients and more recently in adults treated with a special wound-regenerative powder.

8 National Institutes of Health, "Fact Sheet: Regenerative Medicine," http://report.nih.gov/NIHfactsheets/Pdfs/RegenerativeMedicine (NIBIB).pdf (accessed April 16, 2013).

9 Rosemarie Hunziker, "Regenerative Medicine" NIH Fact Sheets, http://report.nih.gov/NIHfactsheets/ViewFactSheet.aspx?csid=62 &key=R (accessed May 18, 2013).

10 Ann Parson, "A Tissue Engineer Sows Cells and Grows Organs," *New York Times*, July 11, 2006, http://www.nytimes.com/2006/07/11 /health/11prof.html?pagewanted=all.

11 Charles A. Vacanti, "The History of Tissue Engineering," *Journal of Cell and Molecular Medicine* 10 (2006): 570.

12 "Regenerative Medicine: Tissue-Engineered Bladder Begins Phase 2 Clinical Trial," McGowan Institute for Regenerative Medicine, http://www.nytimes.com/2006/07/11/health/11prof.html?ex =1310270400&en=799360eaae879b1c&ei=5088&partner=rssnyt &emc=rss (accessed May 18, 2013).

13 http://www.tengion.com/pipeline/overview.cfm (accessed May 18, 2013).

14 Vacanti, "The History of Tissue Engineering," 570.

15 http://www.massgeneral.org/research/researchlab.aspx?id=1129 (accessed May 18, 2013).

16 Henry Fountain, "A First: Organs Tailor-Made with Body's Own Cells," *New York Times*, September 15, 2012, http://www.nytimes .com/2012/09/16/health-research/scientists-make-progress-in-tailor -made-organs.html?pagewanted=all.

17 Henry Fountain, "Groundbreaking Surgery for Girl Born without Windpipe," *New York Times*, April 30, 2013, http://www.nytimes .com/2013/04/30/science/groundbreaking-surgery-for-girl-born -without-windpipe.html?pagewanted=all.

18 Jonathan Lapook and Ryan Jaslow, "Two-Year-Old 'Pioneer' of Stem Cell Trachea Implant Dies," CBS News Online, July 8, 2013, http:// www.cbsnews.com/8301-204_162-57592735/two-year-old-pioneer -of-stem-cell-trachea-transplant-dies/.

19 http://mrmc.amedd.army.mil/index.cfm?pageid=medical_r_and_d .afirm.overview (accessed May 19, 2013).

20 Henry Fountain, "Human Muscle, Regrown on Animal Scaffolding," *New York Times*, September 16, 2012, http://www .nytimes.com/2012/09/17/health/research/human-muscle -regenerated-with-animal-help.html?pagewanted=all.